'Payne's detailed format provides clear information about how to structure activities without being directive; encouraging professionals to use these ideas as guidelines to support or refresh their own skills in exploring the power of dance and movement in groups.'

Suzi Tortora, dance movement therapist, Dancing Dialogue, USA

'This is an excellent introduction to the use of movement and dance in groupwork. It presents theoretical foundations supported by research and the long-time practice of Prof. Payne, as well as helpful structures and procedures.

As a lecturer in MA training programmes for DMP and as a supervisor, I can imagine the smiles of relief of students and professionals in their first stages of their careers when they hold this book in their hands.'

Hilda Wengrower, co-editor of *The Art and Science of Dance/Movement Therapy: Life is Dance* (Routledge, 2009)

'This new edition of *Creative Dance and Movement in Groupwork* Is a welcome and practical resource for dramatherapists and teachers for its attention to the body and what it can tell us. The joy that movement and dance offers is shared in this clearly written new edition and the dramatherapist can explore examples of work within educational, health and community settings.'

Lindsey Fooks, dramatherapist and teacher, Edge Hill University, UK

'As a professional trainer in creative movement and dance, I give a thumbs up to Helen Payne's expanded version of her first book, which was published in 1990. It is an excellent resource for movement activities that can be applicable for the clinical dance movement therapist, as well as practitioners in health, education and social settings.'

Marcia Plevin, psychologist, dance movement therapist, co-founder of Creative Movement and Dance: the Garcìa-Plevin Method

CREATIVE DANCE
AND MOVEMENT IN
GROUPWORK

Creative Dance and Movement in Groupwork continues to explore the link between movement and emotions presented in the first edition of this innovative book. It provides 180 practical activities with a clear rationale for the use of creative dance and movement to enrich therapy or educational programmes.

This book features session plans divided into warm-ups, introductions to themes, development of themes and warm-downs and explores many areas, including developmental movement processes, non-verbal communication, and expression communication. In addition to thoroughly updating the content of the original edition, this timely sourcebook includes new material on creative dance and dance movement psychotherapy, added references throughout and updated resources to reflect the most current knowledge.

Creative Dance and Movement in Groupwork will be an invaluable asset for group leaders wishing to enhance their practice, as well as a starting point for those wishing to learn more about the field. It provides guidance and practical information that is suitable for working with clients of all ages and, for those with a professional or practical interest in the educational, health, recreational or psychotherapeutic use of the arts, this book may act as one of many guiding lights on their journey.

Helen Payne has been an educationalist in special education and is one of the leading pioneers in dance movement psychotherapy (DMP) in the UK and abroad. She was a major innovator of DMP in the UK, leading the development of the professional association and the first research and publications, and has over 100 publications in book, peer-reviewed journal or conference proceeding formats. As well as a small private practice she conducts training in integrative authentic movement and The BodyMind Approach.

Creative Dance and Movement in Groupwork

Second Edition

Helen Payne

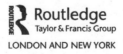
Routledge
Taylor & Francis Group

LONDON AND NEW YORK

Second edition published 2020
by Routledge
2 Park Square, Milton Park, Abingdon, Oxon, OX14 4RN

and by Routledge
52 Vanderbilt Avenue, New York, NY 10017

Routledge is an imprint of the Taylor & Francis Group, an informa business

© 2020 Helen Payne

First edition published by Speechmark Publishing Ltd. 1990
Reprinted by Routledge 2017

British Library Cataloguing-in-Publication Data
A catalogue record for this book is available from the British Library

Library of Congress Cataloging-in-Publication Data
A catalog record has been requested for this book

ISBN: 978-1-138-62581-5 (hbk)
ISBN: 978-1-138-60537-4 (pbk)
ISBN: 978-0-429-45967-2 (ebk)

Typeset in Helvetica
by Swales & Willis, Exeter, Devon, UK

Dedication

This book is dedicated to my mother, Hazel Payne, with blessings, for giving me something of her love for dance.

CONTENTS

About the author

Professor Helen Payne has been one of the leading pioneers in dance movement psychotherapy (DMP) in the UK and abroad. She holds a Ph.D. (London) and an M. Phil. (Manchester) and has over 100 publications in book, peer-reviewed journal or conference proceeding formats. In 1971 she began working in movement and play to develop relationships with adults and children with profound learning difficulties in a hospital setting while attending a specialist physical education course for secondary school teaching. She went on to work with groups in special education, further education, community settings, health and social work. Her further professional studies embrace training in dance, special education, counselling and group analysis. She has held posts on B.Ed., Master's and other postgraduate programmes specialising in DMP.

She is a past programme leader for the first UK-validated postgraduate training in DMP at the University of Hertfordshire, where she also trained art and drama therapists. She then went on to train counsellors at foundation and postgraduate levels. Helen has been a UKCP accredited psychotherapist since 1991 and a senior registered dance movement psychotherapist (ADMP UK) with a small private practice. She regularly acts as principal supervisor and examiner for doctoral candidates and has examined numerous Master's degrees and Ph.D.s. Helen is a professor in Psychotherapy at the University of Hertfordshire and Fellow of ADMP UK with over four decades of practice, training, education and research in the arts therapies, psychotherapy and counselling,

She was a major innovator of DMP in the UK, leading to the development of the professional association, and the first research and publications. She designed and implemented the first foundation and higher education validated postgraduate programmes in DMP. She is founding editor-in-chief for the peer-reviewed *International Journal of Body, Movement and Dance in Psychotherapy* published by Taylor & Francis. Her current research interests include The BodyMind Approach (TBMA), which supports people in learning to self-manage their persistent bodily symptoms for which tests and scans come back negative (medically unexplained symptoms) in primary care; mental health; supervisory practice; and the development of therapeutic presence through the discipline of authentic movement. She teaches and presents nationally and internationally at universities, conferences and professional associations. As well as running a small private practice she conducts training in integrative authentic movement and The BodyMind Approach.

FOREWORD

It was 1993, or around that time. I was looking for directions, personal insights and professional paths. One way forward was to remain a teacher. I was doing a Master's in dance education, after all. Another was to leave the field and get into psychology, a long-standing interest of mine. There was this other field too, dance therapy, neither education nor psychology. Or was it both at the same time? Not sure exactly what it was, curious but scared to leave a path that was expected of me for an area that was new, exciting and so much unknown. My academic tutor, Pat, thought that I needed to explore this new avenue and make up my mind; my interests seem to be relevant. She handed over a few books available in the field, those that were bridging over to therapy. It was early days. Not much was out there, as yet. One of the few publications available was this book, a book one of her own students had written. The author's name was Helen Payne. Activity-based, it spoke to my need to see things in practice. It spoke to my desire to understand how dance could be used in British schools for several different purposes. It allowed me to see how child-centred ideas could be implemented. How ideas from Laban movement analysis could be used so that children could be supported to find their voice and speak their truths in 'body', 'shape', 'space' and 'efforts'. At that time, I had no capacity to value the text as a dance movement therapist, as I was not one yet. The teacher in me, however, was happy with this practical, clear, pedagogically sound text. It offered structures, ideas, games and lots of practical support to people like me, keen and ready to enter a school environment as a dance educator, an educator that wanted to support children to learn and grow. In those days I used it all the time.

It is 2019, and I am a dance movement psychotherapist with qualifications and lengthy experience of working in the field as a clinician, and as an academic. I have written my own book, edited a few more, and published in peer-reviewed journals. I teach dance students and psychotherapists in training. This early publication is almost forgotten. When Helen invited me to write a foreword for its new edition, it reminded me of my first response and admiration for this practical guide for people working with children through movement. In a world where things are constantly changing and text is getting replaced by YouTube videos, this publication retains its charm. It is still equally accessible and interesting. I browse it as an electronic version, as you do these days. I am in Wales in a little yurt surrounded by a wooden decking overseeing a field of bluebells. Charlie, the dog, is with me. He barks at the fresh wind and the sound of the cows lowing at a distance. He seems as happy as I am to be there. As he rolls on the decking with a stick in his mouth, I am thinking I need to join in the play. In the spirit of reviewing the book again, I look at a game that might be relevant for this human/animal dance session. As an experienced practitioner, I can now use the book as inspiration and modify things to suit this unique situation I am in. The book certainly allows me to do this.

Find a few games ... I might use all of them, blending them in unique new ways!

I look at this book again, with fresh eyes, new perspectives and, by now, a different professional identity. I find it fresh and useful, still. I need to remember to include it on the reading list for next year's dance students. I am sure my new Master's students who are interested in using creative methods in psychotherapy will also value it. But, for now, I am going back to playing with Charlie. We both need to move more. With sticks as props or simply with our bodies. In full interactive engagement, in ways that this book certainly supports.

Professor Vicky Karkou, Edge Hill University

PREFACE

This is a brand new, completely updated edition of the first edition entitled *Creative Dance and Movement in Groupwork*. This thoroughly revised and updated second edition, entitled *Creative Dance and Movement in Groupwork*, builds on the first edition, published in 1990, which was reprinted 12 times and translated into at least seven languages. Clearly, it was found to be of immense support as a sourcebook for facilitating creative dance and movement with a range of people with different needs in groups, whether for dance movement psychotherapy (DMP) or as employed by professional practitioners in health, community, social care and educational settings. This edition clarifies these different and distinct approaches. The activities can be flexible to suit different intentions, goals, approaches, settings and populations. I developed some of the activities from my practice with children, adolescents and adults with multiple difficulties, limited receptive and expressive language, and behavioural, intellectual and/or physical disabilities. Communication was often problematic. Individual styles were hard to understand sometimes. Due to my background in movement and dance I started to improvise in movement as a way for clients/patients to communicate feelings and thoughts. They were invited to follow my movement as well as initiate and lead the movement conversations. Sometimes sessions included music, sometimes singing, sometimes percussion. This is how my journey into DMP began.

It should be noted that the term 'dance movement psychotherapy' is employed in the UK. In the USA the profession is referred to as 'dance/movement therapy' or 'dance therapy', in Europe it is 'dance movement therapy' (as previously in the UK) and in India 'creative movement therapy' is used. Since the book is published in the UK it will use dance movement psychotherapy (DMP).

In addition to providing a thoroughly expanded and updated version of the previously published content, this timely sourcebook includes new material on DMP, added references throughout and updated resources in Section 4 to reflect the most current knowledge.

Who is the book for?

This book is for anyone offering creative dance and movement groupwork whether in educational, health or community settings. It is especially aimed at teachers, many of whom will be in special education or engaged in inclusive education; community dance workers/practitioners delivering groups in health, education and social settings; and dance movement psychotherapists working with groups in health and educational contexts.

The application of creative dance and movement in groupwork in education (particularly special education), health, and social and community settings is increasing rapidly by all of the above professionals. Additionally, the growing obesity and mental health conditions in current society, especially for children and young people, mean regular movement-based creative activity is even more important. Many people are new to this application and want to establish some starting-points before using creative dance and movement; and those who have begun may be seeking to reflect on and develop their practice.

The book is also written for people without specialist knowledge of creative dance and movement in groupwork who are looking for such starting-points. If you have a professional or practical interest in the educational, health, recreational or psychotherapeutic use of the arts, this book may act as one of many guiding lights on your journey.

This book is the only reference book on creative dance and movement giving practical examples and resources to a wide range of practitioners from education, community performance, therapeutic recreation, health and psychotherapy fields.

The book is also intended to be a helpful reference guide for professional practitioners in DMP already familiar with facilitating groups. For those who (like me) sometimes feel helpless when working with particularly challenging, disturbed or disabled groups, this book can provide new energy and empowerment; you can do something!

The aims of the book

This is a practical book to refer to frequently: not a textbook or something to be read once from cover to cover, and certainly not an instruction manual. It gives essential information and guidance, but if your aim is to further your skills in this medium you are advised to attend professional training courses and read widely (see Section 4); reading this book will definitely not make you a dance movement psychotherapist.

Whilst the book is essentially a source of activities, it also emphasises the need to reflect on the work done. I hope, therefore, that use of the activities will be complemented by reference to the other sections of the book. However, the emphasis is on 'good enough' practice at all times and the guidelines presented aim to encourage you to experiment with activities and to act as a springboard for your own ideas.

It is also important to say that this is not a 'how-to-do-it' manual; it neither defines a correct procedure for using creative dance and movement nor provides a blueprint for successful work with your own groups. There is no simple 'right way' to practice that guarantees the achievement of goals. This may be valid when applied to the assembly of objects, for example, although the following quotation casts doubt even on that:

> ... what's really angering about instructions of this sort is that they imply there's only one way to put this rotisserie together—their way. And that presumption wipes out all creativity. Actually there are hundreds of ways to put the rotisserie together and when they make you follow just one way without showing you the overall problem the instructions become hard to follow in such a way as not to make mistakes. You lose feeling for the work. And not only that, it's very unlikely that they've told you the best way.
>
> (Pirsig, 1976, 160)

In work involving human relations, self-awareness and developmental processes, the elements of creativity and feeling that Pirsig refers to are of even greater significance. Leading groups is a matter of finding ways of working with relationships and problems that are unique to each group, leader and setting. As in many complex situations, much depends on how information such as that provided in this book is understood and on how well it is adapted. In each situation there are many opportunities and possible pitfalls.

My hope is that this book will give groupwork practitioners and psychotherapists a continued feel for their work and a new confidence in their own way of doing things. If your response, when reading it or applying it to practice, is 'That's right, that's what I'm doing' or 'That's what I wanted to do', then this hope will have been fulfilled. In conclusion, *Creative Dance and Movement in Groupwork* aims to help you to arrive at sound decisions on how to proceed, decisions about which you feel good and which use your own creativity.

The book's contents

The book is written in four sections:

Section 1 gives a brief description of the history and background of movement and dance work. The roles of the dance and movement groupwork practitioner in relation to the dance movement psychotherapist are articulated. This is the section to read if you want to know how creative dance and movement has come to be used in treatment and rehabilitation, and why and how it is of value.

Section 2 outlines the principles of movement, including developmental movement and Rudolf Laban's movement categorisation on which creative dance and movement is based. This provides a brief outline of the main theoretical models and tools of creative dance and movement. The section also gives practical advice on the planning, development and evaluation of programmes of dance and movement.

Section 3, which constitutes both the bulk and the heart of the book, describes activities that have been found to be workable with groups of children, adolescents and adults in a variety of settings. Although written from reflections of groupwork practice, many of these activities can be undertaken in individual work. Indeed, I have tested them myself within one-to-one practice. A core principle of the book is that action and evaluation proceed simultaneously, so that most activities incorporate suggestions for future development. The activities are open to discussion and modification, to be experimented with and improved upon by you. Some activities can be reviewed in discussion time within the group, further promoting levels of insight and understanding for individuals.

Section 4 gives further information, such as references, a glossary of terms, training courses and other helpful addresses.

Finally, no programme of creative dance and movement can exist in isolation; it needs to relate to the specific problems and strengths of the population you are working with and to the approach of the setting. Nor can a programme exist outside you; what you contribute both personally and professionally will shape the programme's nature and success.

ACKNOWLEDGEMENTS[1]

There are many people I would like to thank for their support and inspiration throughout my life, unfortunately far too many to mention by name here. I would, however, like to say a special thank you to all the clients and patients in the various hospitals, clinics, special schools and community homes, without whom this book could not have come to fruition. They continue to initiate me and to teach me on my journey.

1 This book is based on a booklet written by the author in 1982, entitled *Stepping In,* and published by the Association for Dance Movement Therapy: ISBN 0 951025 60 0 (limited to 100 copies).

BACKGROUND

Introduction

Dance has been part of human life throughout the ages, performed to celebrate, for example, births, marriages, harvests and wars (Sachs, 1937). People dance as naturally as they play, court, feed or fight and dance is often used to express those functions. Throughout the world dance is part of our rituals (see Glossary) and our heritage. In the UK *The Gulbenkian Dance Report* (1980) defined dance as part of the history of human movement, part of the history of human culture, and part of the history of human communication.

Growth, health and creativity are often seen to be interrelated, the potential for all being present in human beings. Improvisation and re-enactment, through dance, of earlier experience, can help to release tension and aid self-expression and integration. In our society, where there is perhaps a declining emphasis on physical work or action, energy is often repressed; hence the popular need for physical outlets such as the leisure pursuits of aerobics and jogging.

A recent study by Tarr, Launay and Dunbar (2016) demonstrated that the effects of dancing together in synchrony and with exertion reduced pain and increased a sense of belonging (social bonding). In a study on the perceived benefits of dancing on wellness from an 'arts in health' perspective, quantitative and qualitative analysis revealed that dancing has potential positive benefits on well-being. Benefits related to emotional as well as physical, social and spiritual dimensions. In addition, the positive benefits were also linked to self-esteem and coping strategies (Murcia, Kreutz, Clift and Bongard, 2010). Argentine tango and mixed-genre therapeutic dancing classes accompanied by home programmes are feasible and safe for people in the early to mid-stages of Parkinson's disease, according to a study by Rocha, Aguiar,

McClelland and Morris (2018). Gomes, Menezes and Oliveira (2014) found from their meta-analysis of dance therapy with patients with chronic heart failure that dance therapy should be considered for inclusion in cardiac rehabilitation as it improves exercise- and health-related quality of life.

Earlier research (for example, Doyne et al., 1987) has demonstrated that this action of physical doing helps to release tension and reduce depression. Dance and movement are active, dynamic, body-based, expressive and communicative media; the build-up of adrenalin can be dispersed and aggression, rigidity and apathy can be discharged in a socially acceptable manner. To dance out anger or joy, love or sadness enhances the individual's ability to express these affects. Inaction and depression are often synonymous; the creative act of moving alone or with others can enable an integration of mind, body and spirit.

An early study by Puretz (1978) compared the effects of dance and physical education on the self-concept of disadvantaged girls. There was a significant increase in the dance subjects' self-concept. In another study, May, Wexler, Falkin and Schoop (1978), schizophrenics were shown to benefit from group dance movement therapy, and later studies for this population have found dance movement therapy to reduce negative effects (Röhricht and Priebe, 2006). Leste and Rust (1984) studied the effects of modern dance on anxiety with subjects in further education. Their results indicated a statistically significant drop in scores for anxiety levels in the experimental group in comparison to the music therapy and physical education control groups.

The effects of dance movement psychotherapy (DMP) interventions and the therapeutic use of dance were studied in a meta-analysis of research conducted over the past 20 years by Koch, Kuntz, Lykou and Cruz (2014). This showed moderate effects for quality of life and clinical outcomes (depression, anxiety) and yielded small but consistent effects for improvement of well-being, mood, affect and body image. The analysis included the effects of 23 evidence-based primary studies for 15 populations (N = 1078).

There are significantly more studies demonstrating the positive outcomes of dance movement (psycho)therapy (DMP) on numerous populations (for details see Koch and Brauninger, 2006; Goodill, 2016; Buse, Sarikaya and Colucci, 2017). Cochrane reviews for DMP and dementia (Karkou and Meekums, 2014), and for depression (Meekums, Karkou and Nelson, 2012) have been conducted additionally (for further details on UK research please see www.admp.org.uk).

Other areas of considerable research have been in the fields of body image, movement in space and proximetrics (the body in space and in relationships), for example, early studies of the proximity-seeking behaviour of infants and children towards their mother after a period of separation (Heinicke and Westheimer, 1966). More recently there has been research relevant to the practice of creative dance and movement, from fields such as neuroscience (Gallese, Keysers and Rizzolatti, 2004; Damasio, 2010), psychiatry and psychotherapy (Siegel, 2012), infant research (Trevarthen, 2003), anthropology (Cozolino, 2006) and in attunement in early attachment and interpersonal neurobiology (Schore, 2012; Trevarthen and Delafield-Butt, 2013). Siegel (2012) states:

> Parents attune to the subtle changes in the baby's state of arousal, revealed as the vitality affect, not merely the categorical affect that the infant may be expressing. In fact, this expression of internal state through vitality affects the primary mode of communication between an infant and a caregiver during the early years of life. (p. 154)

Physiological motor developmental patterns need examining alongside affective, cognitive and social development. Reaching out, for example, will enable the infant to grasp an object and pull it towards themselves. This experience will also give the infant a sense of control, mastery and capacity to affect their environment (agency). The movements become 'more purposeful' as noted by Sherborne (2001, p. 64). Movement meets functional needs, such as grasping a cup of water, as well as the expression of thoughts and feelings, linking the self with others/the environment. Shared movement enables communication of shared social meaning. The infant opens their arms to their caregiver who reaches down to pick them up.

Touch and rhythm can provide a holding container, as can music and vocal sounds. Scholgler and Trevarthen (2007) found connections between singing, dancing and attunement reflecting interpersonal communications. Self-regulation through empathic attunement can be enhanced when clients express rhythmic sound and movement in the psychotherapeutic context. This shared dance (Samaritter and Payne, 2017) does not need to be contained verbally, although verbal reflection towards the end of sessions is encouraged for those able to make use of it. Meaning-making arising from embodied presence in the movement moment is created whenever there is synchrony and/or empathic attunement. Rhythm in movement, for example, provides a safe, non-verbal platform for structuring the interaction between participants, the safety of the rhythm supporting the process of separation and differentiation versus unity and connectedness. The predictability of rhythm forms the basis for a trusting relationship. It is connected to attunement and the baby's safety in the womb from synchronicity with the mother, e.g. regular pulse, heartbeat and mother's breathing patterns, walking and speaking. Life in the mother's womb is shaped by auditory, vibratory, tactile, proprioceptive and kinaesthetic stimuli to provide early attunement. The tone of voice, pitch and variation make a connection with the infant that is important for the attachment process. The rhythm of nursery rhymes reflects the heartbeat.

Touch, via the physical holding of the primary caregiver, and the quality and ways in which the infant is handled, can continue the previous shared rhythms. Physical holding gives sensory input, which in turn gives a sense of self as separate, as the infant becomes more differentiated from the other through the act of being held (Winnicott, 1971). Confidence, sensitivity, tentativeness, fearfulness etc. are communicated through touch. The physical contact experienced by someone physically in need of care tends to be functional, hence a more formal relationship with any carer will develop. Appropriate touch within movement group-work can be introduced safely to promote a sensitive, reciprocal relationship. Touch can emerge spontaneously between people in the group during creative movement practices as well, so it is important to monitor this systematically to ensure it is safe and appropriate. Additionally, it is important to acknowledge that touch can stimulate previous unwanted experiences (such as physical or sexual abuse) for some people as well as their previous background of being held.

The mirror neuron system, next to the motor area in the brain, has a role in the development of empathic attunement (Gallese, Keysers and Rizzolatti, 2004). By seeing and mirroring 'as if' experiencing other people's physical actions, attunement and empathy in interpersonal relationships are developed. Embodied simulation (Gallese and Sinigaglia, 2011a, 2011b) is where we can simulate the intentions behind the action/s of another (see Payne, 2017a for details of how this can apply to the processes in Laban movement analysis (LMA) and authentic movement). This attunement then 'creates emotional resonance' with the other (Siegel, 2007, p. 167). Furthermore, the bridge between bodily sensation (employed frequently in creative dance and movement practices) and empathy are the mirror neurons. Emotional responses are elicited in the observer from postures, gestures, facial expressions and socially meaningful movements, which is the bottom-up neurological basis for the social nature of humans. Healthy attachment grounded in interpersonal connection with a significant other is the basis for cognition (Trevarthen, 2003; Siegel, 2012).

Neuroscience shows us that cognitions and emotions are embodied and modal (Shapiro, 2011), and that concepts partially originate in the subjective experience anchored in the body and simulated by the activation of corresponding aspects of such experiences. Schore (2012) supports the idea that emotional content of interpersonal communication can be reframed by stimulating the pre-linguistic pathways in the right brain and limbic system, which can be triggered by intentional movement as in dance. The immediacy of this spontaneous movement improvisation can mirror the earliest relationship. Damasio (2010) concurs that feelings are held in the body and brain networks rather than solely cerebrally. The arts, he says, are rooted in biology and the human body yet can elevate humans to heights in thought and feelings, compensating for emotional imbalances such as grief, anger, fear or desire. Consequently, the argument has been made that the arts can offer transformation to mental health and well-being (for further discussion on the application to DMP of this research please see Payne, 2017b).

creative dance and movement do not rely so heavily, as do verbal methods, on linguistic or intellectual capacities for inter- and intrapersonal exploration. Since dance can derive from an inner, spontaneous stimulus without the aid of music, as well as evolving from learning steps and 'dancing to music', it provides an ideal vehicle for change, being expressive and communicative in its performance. creative dance and movement in this context can thus be viewed as embodied interpersonal intentionality and non-functional, ideal for groups! This dynamic between people moving in a group can support recreational and educational objectives as well as psychotherapeutic change.

Historical development

The systematic use of dance and movement in treatment of mental/emotional health and well-being with various populations, both in the UK and the USA, dates back over three quarters of a century. To some extent this development in the UK has been separate from that in the USA, although these two strands have become more closely connected over time.

The UK has long had a tradition of including creative dance as a core educational discipline, especially at primary school level. Recognition of the potential for rehabilitation and therapy through dance and movement experiences began in the UK in the 1940s, although very little was written about the work at that time.

A significant figure in the development of modern dance in Europe and creative dance in the UK educational system was Rudolf von Laban (1879–1958) due to his presence in Manchester. His contribution included the systematic categorisation of movement both for writing down dances (Labanotation) (Hutchinson, 1970) and a taxonomy of human movement for movement observation (LMA) (North, 1972; Moore, 2009). Adrian (2008) and Newlove (1993) show how Laban's movement analysis was applied to the training of actors for character development, helping them to move their bodies in a way that reflects feelings (Laban, 1971, 1975). His theory is core to the Sesame approach to drama and movement, which integrates touch, sound, story-telling, play and Jungian psychology to explore metaphor supporting transformation in therapy. The author completed part of the Sesame programme where she worked with Audrey Wethered (1973), a Jungian analyst who studied individually with Laban. Later she trained with another of Laban's students, Marion North (1972) and with Laban's partner, Lisa Ullman.

In DMP, LMA enables the therapist to use movement observations as both a diagnostic and an assessment element in the work. Laban's analysis and categorisation of movement has added to the other bodies of literature on non-verbal communication. His early thinking on movement therapy is described in an article (1983) written in 1949 when he was working with patients in Exeter. One of Laban's students, Warren Lamb, added to the analysis a category focusing on shape (Lamb and Watson, 1979), which evolved out of his work in management training.

Following Laban's analysis of movement and contribution to dance in education, his students and others began to promote the use of dance and movement in treatment and therapeutic contexts. For example, Laban students Veronica Sherborne (1974, 2001) and Wethered (and Gardner) (1986) used Laban's contribution as far back as the 1940s for children with severe learning difficulties and adults hospitalised for mental health conditions respectively. Theorists such as North (1972) later added to his ideas, correlating movement with personality traits. Others such as Bainbridge, Duddington, Collingdon and Gardner (1953) used creative dance in psychiatry and Oliver (1968, 1975) had success employing dance in hospitals and schools for people with a cognitive impairment.

In the 1950s education authorities such as the then West Riding authority and Manchester authority pioneered the use of Laban's work in their education of teachers and in their primary and secondary schools. They trained primary and specialist secondary teachers of physical education in the application of his ideas to movement and dance education, which stressed creativity and groupwork approaches.

Soon all education authorities were using Laban's principles in their dance and movement education programmes. The child-centred educational philosophy in England at that time helped in the fostering of the work, which was endorsed by the Department of Education and Science (Foster, 1977) and called 'modern educational dance' (Laban, 1971).

Although Laban was a gifted thinker and teacher and had a profound effect on the history and development of creative dance in the UK, the status of his theories has been criticised by, for example, Gordon Curl as early as 1967, and by others later. One major source of contention is that some of Laban's writings speak of movement in formal geometrical and arbitrary cosmological terms and do not acknowledge that movement takes place in phenomenal space, within a context. Thus, there is scepticism about ascribing expressive meanings to movement, which is not contextualised or qualitatively based, by reference to a preconceived cosmological theory.

The USA saw the earlier development of a specific therapy using dance and movement, together with the formation of a professional association, the American Dance Therapy Association (ADTA), in 1966. The American literature of the 1960s and 1970s relates the pioneering dance movement therapists' perceptions of the therapeutic process (Chace, 1975). Dance and movement experiences were found to help groups of mentally ill and 'handicapped' people in a variety of ways; however, the practice in general stemmed from modern dance as a performance art as opposed to Laban dance.

In the UK since the 1960s, in isolated pockets, physical educators, special educators, dance educators and artists, social workers, nurses, psychologists, physiotherapists, occupational therapists and others have explored these media with populations (see Glossary) such as psychiatric patients, people with a learning difference, individuals on the autistic spectrum, young offenders, the elderly, substance misusers and children at risk.

Dance movement psychotherapists in the UK have defined professional boundaries and a basis for the work is becoming more and more established due to increased research and publications. However, the profession has developed later than the other arts therapies in the UK and dance/movement therapy[1] in the USA. This has been the result of, for example, practitioners working in isolation, and a lack of written and published evidence of practice.

The Association for Dance Movement Therapy was formally established in 1982 (Payne, 1983, 1985). It has since been renamed The Association for Dance Movement Psycho-therapy (ADMP UK) (www.admp.org.uk) and registered members can apply to become accredited by the United Kingdom Council of Psychotherapy as dance movement psychotherapists, one of the two national bodies for accrediting psychotherapists from a number of orientations. Among the aims of ADMP UK are registration of members, accreditation of postgraduate training and education in dance movement psychotherapy, promotion of the profession and the provision of a shared focal point for practitioners in the field. Despite the enormous energy and activity to develop the field, employment opportunities remain the remit of qualified practitioners who have to create their own work, whether freelance/sessional, part time, as an aspect of another role or in private practice. The new government initiative for schools to be increasingly responsible for mental health and well-being may offer more possibilities for employment in the arts therapies, however.

Dance as movement and dance as performance art

Everyone has a general idea of dance as an art form. For those people relatively new to the field it may be useful to set out the differences between the use of dance as an art form and the use of dance as movement in psychotherapy. DMP grew out of the use of dance and movement with special needs groups but has since become more distinct. It is important to make some of these distinctions clear for those people intending to use this book.

Something that may be puzzling for those new to the arts therapies, but which is an issue of considerable significance for the professions, is the distinction between practitioners working as teachers or artists with special needs groups—whose work nonetheless may be therapeutic—and practitioners working as psychotherapists with those same populations. In the UK field of dance and movement, the former was exemplified by early pioneers such as Wolfgang Stange and his calisthenics with people with learning differences (then termed mentally handicapped) and Gina Levete (1985), and the latter by those such as Payne (1979, 1984, 1992, 2006a, 2017b) and Meekums (1987, 2002). Each field has provided new ideas and research.

Movement and creativity are the vehicle for both fields, with its raw materials of the body, time, space, and energy or force. However, the intentions will be different. When using dance as art it may focus on, for example, perform-ance, exercise or educational aims. It is the context and underlying assumptions that determine such aims.

Dance as movement is the conceptual approach used in DMP. It bypasses any exercise or aesthetic aspects inherent in the art of dance; rather its nature is explained in psychotherapeutic, psychological, sociological and/or historical terms. DMP in the UK is a development of the original 'movement' approach to dance common in the 1960s, which then formed the basis for the 'human movement studies' model of the mid-1970s. Then, dance was one example of a movement form amongst many. This is the context for adopting the term 'dance move-ment *psycho*therapy' in the UK, in contrast to the term 'dance therapy' or 'dance/movement therapy', which refers to either dance or movement, used in the USA. It is interesting to note the professional association ADTA in the USA defines the term dance/movement therapy (DMT) as 'a psychotherapeutic approach'. Professionals have to be accredited as counsellors in order to practice DMT, however the term 'psychotherapy' is not reflected in their terminology for the profession.

The 1980s saw dance grow as a performance art extending into educational and community contexts as well as with special needs groups. Dance as performance art offers technique and choreography and these relate to modern dance as developed in the performance art for the theatre. When using dance as a performance art, however, a particular style of movement technique is employed. The form and the technique are derived from a specific body-based training in a style such as ballet, Cunningham, Haw-kins, Limon or Graham (Cohen, 1966).

Laban's approach, used by therapists and others, emphasises creative dance in which movement is self-generated and linked together, so forming the dance. The components are employed by the mover or therapist for expression or intervention. In this area of creative dance, the main points of interest might be, for example, move-ment qualities, or the relationships between people through body activity in the dance and the use it makes of space.

The orientation towards either dance as movement or dance as art influences the aims and nature of the session, methods for development, and evaluation procedures; this will be true whether the session is for psychotherapy, edu-cation, performance or some other aim. During creative dance, any form and style present are those the individual chooses to use. Improvisation can lead to a depth in feeling commensurate with the movement process. The mover could begin to work with, for example, reclaiming or recon-necting with specific parts of their body: by becoming more self-aware they may acknowledge imperfections or exert a more positive control over their bodies.

The major difference between dance as a performance art and dance as movement in psychotherapy lies in the basic theory. The central principle of DMP is that a significant and powerful connection exists between motion and emotion, an interrelationship between body and mind. The role of the psychotherapist is to give attention to the mover, helping them to explore this connection in their own life and experience, with the aim of healing themselves and enriching the relationship between physical and psycho-emotional elements. This movement process is a dance, but as such it does not aim to make 'art', increase exercise or to use dance for performance, although these might be spin-offs. The approach to, and context of, that dance are significantly different.

This central principle is grounded in knowledge about child development. Long before an infant understands verbal communications or responds to visual cues, it feels the subtleties of the mother's physical attentions and of its own movement. These early memories are pre-verbal, since the nervous system is insufficiently developed for the storage of verbal information. The early mother–infant relationship is a symbiotic phase, one of memories pre-verbally stored in the body. Through kinaesthetic sensations, particularly in holding and handling by the mother, the body image, a sense of self and the mind's structure emerge.

There are stage-specific actions that occur throughout the normal development of a child; these include grasping, rolling, rocking, creeping, throwing, crawling, standing, falling, balancing, walking, running, skipping and jumping. Attitudes of family members towards these actions may need to be identified and worked with to free the person from inhibitions experienced in childhood because of, say, negative parental attitudes towards climbing. Furthermore, blocks to healthy development can occur due to abuse, trauma and/or insecure attachment, which can manifest in movement expression.

Any movement not experienced at the appropriate stage of development because of attitudes or restrictions may be experienced at a later stage, even in an adult body. Over-keen parenting can also damage normal development as with, for example, pushing a child to walk before crawling has been consolidated. These 'lost' experiences of motoric development can be physicalised through specific structures: for example, sitting to turning to crawling to sitting sequences. The adult may eventually recapture some of the perceptual and emotional processes accompanying such a stage. Therefore, a knowledge of the fundamental physical stages in infant–child development can be useful to those of us working with, for example, developmentally delayed groups or those who have become impoverished at a particular stage, for whatever reason.

Thus, there are some basic differences between dance performance, creative dance and DMP; while dance performance and creative dance, like sport, may have therapeutic effects, it does not constitute a psychotherapy in itself because it does not pursue systematically psychotherapeutic goals such as the integration of conscious and unconscious experience. DMP has a clear basis for its psychotherapeutic value. Practitioners trained in dance as performance with a specific technique can develop into dance movement psychotherapists; indeed, some early therapists were typically so trained, although more so in the USA than in the UK. What is important is that, in DMP, dance skills/technique and education and/or performance cease to be the main aims of the work.

The role of the dance and movement practitioner in relation to the dance movement psychotherapist

This issue needs to be addressed when groupwork practitioners are working in the field without a formal training in DMP. All practitioners, whether in creative dance and movement in groupwork or dance movement psychotherapists facilitating groups, need to ensure their practice is within the limitations of their training and qualifications. In DMP, registered membership with the professional association is now a requirement for a license to practice.

Stickley and Clift (2017) delineate some useful research, theory and practice understanding from the impact of the arts in mental health and chronic pain to community-based activity through arts therapies and considerations around making the economic case.

Fancourt (2017) gives guidance for arts in health practitioners in designing and researching interventions and Clift and Camic (2015) in an international handbook present a thorough overview of the field of arts in health, outlining very helpful practices, research and theory from a global perspective. These may help clarify some of the issues between creative dance and movement as employed for well-being in health, education and recreation in the community, and creative dance and movement as a form of psychotherapy. It is important to make this clarification of intentions and context, so that employers, clients and patients are aware of any implications (for example, ethical issues).

The practitioner, who may have training in teaching, dance, occupational therapy, groupwork or another related area, has a complementary role to that of the dance movement psychotherapist. Both work with individuals of all ages who have social, emotional, sensory, cognitive and physical problems (some of these problems are present together). Both are employed to work with individuals and groups by agencies such as psychiatric hospitals, clinics, day care services, community health centres, special schools or prisons. Both can act as consultants and may engage in research, and both need to identify their overall aims for their groups, whether creative, educational or therapeutic.

Experience of working with special needs groups in dance and movement is valuable for those wishing to train as dance movement psychotherapists. Each role will be examined individually next.

The creative dance and movement practitioner

Practitioners such as qualified physical educators, dance teachers or dance artists aim to give opportunities in the media of dance and movement to special needs groups, who would otherwise normally be excluded from such experiences. The relationship is 'teacher to student', rather than 'therapist to client', and the contract is different from psychotherapy: the emphasis is on enjoyment, exercise, aesthetic pleasure and education, such as knowledge and understanding of, and skills in, dance and/or movement. The experiences on offer may include visits to dance performances; undertaking a series of classes with a dance company, leading to a final performance in the establishment; and choreographic workshops with a group and their teachers, which again may help a group to perform dances in the hospital or school and so on. Practitioners using dance and movement may also include people with a disability as equal partners in classes and as dance performers.

The social prescribing initiative in the UK (Bickerdike et al., 2017; Department of Health and Social Care, 2018) is a means of enabling GPs, nurses and other primary care professionals to refer people to a range of local, non-clinical services to improve their health and well-being. Creative dance and movement groups can be conducted within this remit by dance artists and other practitioners with an interest in supporting vulnerable people who can be referred to community-based creative movement/dance classes. Similarly, it is widely acknowledged now that the arts and creativity can positively impact health and well-being.

The arts in health movement (part of The Royal Society of Public Health) provides a platform for developing dance and creative movement programmes for a large cohort of the population, again via the arts on prescription system (for more details see www.networks.nhs.uk/nhs-networks/arts-in-healthcare). For an example, see Arts and Minds (www.artsandminds.org.uk/projects/arts-on-prescription/).

Through such experiences the senses may be heightened, and a potential discovered. Physical and perceptual skills may be fostered, and aspects such as body awareness, self-image, intuition and the integration of thought and emotions may be enhanced. These are all important outcomes, but the modification of symptoms and/or engagement with the emotional life of the client is not the primary purpose for this type of practitioner. Rather, they seek to develop opportunities for educating and enriching lives and to create positive achievements. Their aim is to offer dance as an art form or performance (not necessarily public), which is often an outcome of their work.

The dance movement psychotherapist

The major role of the dance movement psychotherapist is to complement that of the creative dance and movement practitioner. They aim to bring about, with someone whose development has been arrested or has taken an abnormal path, durable, positive change in the direction of physical, emotional and social well-being, or to help a person to more fully achieve their potential.

The dance or movement activity and any resulting formed dance becomes the method for diagnosis and further psycho-therapeutic intervention, or a vehicle for supporting the health of the client. The dance movement psychotherapist, educated in the human sciences (including psychotherapy), creative dance and movement forms, is committed to the psycho-therapeutic use of dance and creative movement as a discipline to further the person's emotional growth and psychological and social integration. They select from their wide-ranging psychotherapy, dance, movement and observa-tion skills to enable contact with otherwise isolated and diffi-cult client groups. They work in mental health treatment, and rehabilitative and special educational settings. They plan and evaluate sessions and work towards agreed therapeutic goals, often within a multidisciplinary team. Sometimes this practice takes place as a prerequisite for those clients unable to benefit from the dance practitioner's input, or alongside their work. In common with the other arts therapies, an important dimension of DMP is that it offers simultaneous access to both feeling and symbolic levels of human experience.

Professional dance movement psychotherapists have a postgraduate training (see Section 4), which includes a range of dance and movement skills, core humanistic or integrative psychotherapy knowledge, understanding and skills, clinical studies, anatomy and physiology, anthropology, human development, observation of move-ment, supervised clinical practice, and research, assess-ment and evaluation skills. They are regularly supervised for practice in at least two different settings and have experienced their own psychotherapy in a relevant orientation.

These two types of practitioner are therefore not mutu-ally exclusive; they do, however, have different priorities and, in consequence, training and education, policy-makers and employers need to acknowledge these differences. It is important that any contract should clearly stipulate if the proposed group is to be psychotherapy, educational, performance, recreational etc.

A more detailed description of the process of DMP now follows.

Dance movement psychotherapy: the mode of working

During DMP, unconsciously derived movement responses can elicit the associated recall and re-enactment of early phenomena, making conscious the imprint of feelings that may be re-experienced and acknowledged at a different level of consciousness.

People can engage deeply in this process through functioning at a non-verbal level, with movement as the medium. Creative dance improvisations and unconscious free associational movement are fundamental to this form of therapy, whether it takes place individually or in groups. By employing expressive approaches such as in Laban's methods and facilitating play in movement and sensory processes, re-experiencing and symbolic enactment enable the pre-verbal experience, however deeply buried, to become explicit.

The client (or patient), not the psychotherapist, is the one who can create change, although the therapist needs to believe in the client's ability to do so. Clients may be encouraged to work in one of two ways during sessions; both ways are spontaneous, self-initiated and self-directed. The first is an 'outside-in', the second an 'inside-out' approach. Improvisation requires a spontaneity of activity, something many groups find difficult. Movement can stir the feelings, just as feelings can stir and be reflected in movement. A cautious approach, with carefully selected activities, will be demanded before some groups are confident enough to improvise.

In the first approach (outside-in) the psychotherapist sets a theme and offers music and a movement game or a structure, and the group works within that. Movement is often with eyes open and the movement relates to an actual person or object; it aids awareness of emotional patterns that group members establish with others in their immediate environment. The Chacian Circle developed by Marian Chace (Chaiklin, 1975) in the USA might be an example of this approach.

The second approach (inside-out) involves the group in self-initiated movements that arise out of interactions, feelings and opportunities created in the session for individual work, such as identifying a physical symptom and moving 'as if ... ' This is often done with eyes closed (opening them at intervals to keep an orientation in the room) and the movement relates only to the internal process as it is being experienced, often as a pre-conscious state. With this second approach, the individuals in the group move from feelings, sensations, thoughts or images that emerge spontaneously from within themselves, rather than to any suggestions from the psychotherapist. These images are generated from either bodily-based feelings, sensations or the spontaneous movements themselves; the images emerge into awareness and by so doing can help to identify the experience of the mover. This method is more appropriate for 'neurotic' than 'psychotic' client groups, since it requires the capacity to bear the tension of opposites (to open fully to the unconscious while maintaining a strong conscious standpoint).

These pre-verbal experiences may then be shared at a verbal level if appropriate, transforming body-felt experiences into thoughts and words (externalising them to others). The changing self may be reflected in the body image, which needs to be moved rather than talked through in order to give the individual feedback at the pre-verbal level from their own body and movement. However, verbalisation at the right time can be a supportive aspect of the process, as long as it is not overused. The reality orientation of the body work needs to be returned to after such dialogue. Feedback from others helps to encourage new body-felt relationships. Alternatively, different media can be used; for example, sometimes by using drawing or sound-making the movement process can be clarified. To begin to expose the self in moving action can be difficult for some groups, or some individuals in the group; simply being in the space with the group, or the expressing of the 'non-movement' issue through verbal acknowledgement may be major achievements. With other groups the continued need to move all the time may be a defense or resistance to being still, talking or reflecting. This approach is akin to the discipline of authentic movement developed by Whitehouse, Chodorow and Adler cited in Pallaro (1999, 2007). For further details of this approach see Chodorow (1991); Adler (2002) and Payne (2006b).

Taking responsibility for one's movement action involves taking responsibility for the self in action and the feelings one has in the process. This can result in a will to change. After acknowledging (owning) the feeling and expressing it in the 'dance', some communication can then develop within the inner world of the client and finally in the outer world, from self to other.

The area of dance movement as psychotherapy is no longer embryonic, it has been found to be effective and meaningful for a variety of client groups and grown significantly since 1990 when the first edition of this book was published. For example, there are several academic postgraduate training programmes across the UK now (whereas in 1988 when the first edition of this book was being written there was only one UK validated programme), and also many more in Europe and the rest of the world. Globally, additional books have been produced, both sole-author and edited, another journal *Body, Movement and Dance in Psychotherapy*, published by Taylor & Francis, was launched in 2006, and further research has been undertaken, although much more research is required. The UK professional association is now approaching its 40th year. There have been many attainments since its formation. One particular attainment is the achievement of accreditation as dance movement *psycho*therapists for registered members through one of the two major bodies overseeing professional accreditation of psychotherapists—the United Kingdom Council for Psychotherapy, via the Humanistic and Integrative Psychotherapy College.

A new European professional association has been formed with membership from almost all professional associations in Europe. It holds conferences bi-annually, and registers training programmes. Furthermore, countries worldwide are beginning their own professional associations and training. There is talk of a world alliance for DMT being formed in the future.

Training in dance movement psychotherapy

The essence of DMP lies in the process rather than the technique. How it is used will depend on your talents in the art of movement and dance as well as the receptivity of the client to dance and movement. It is crucial that you have the capacity to attend, hear and listen to the client's communications in the dance or movement as well as to verbalisation.

If you are interested in developing your talents in dance and movement and in responding in depth to clients in this medium as a dance movement psychotherapist, then a professional academic postgraduate training course is imperative (please see Section 4 for programmes around the world). Anyone who is working with groups, is qualified in one of the helping professions and/or psychology or other relevant profession such as teaching, and/or has extended training or experience in dance and movement could consider entering postgraduate training in DMP. In addition, there are other types of training at various levels, both non-validated and validated by various bodies, and self-financing, available in the UK and abroad. Some examples are featured in Section 4 of this volume.

Conclusion

This section has given a brief introduction to the part creative dance and movement experiences play in treatment and rehabilitation. Wounds can never heal completely; a person always reflects the fact of having been healed or healing, and dance and movement are not a panacea, certain to produce growth, health or cure. However, the group who have danced together will have been assisted towards, for example, becoming more cohesive, more responsive, more aware of their choices and more courageous.

The aim of dance and movement work is not simply to evoke or reflect feelings, but to encourage the client to begin to feel in expressive action. Working towards acknowledging the body more and reawakening the initial life force enables people to become participants in their own change process.

Finally, as practitioners and dance movement psychotherapists, our own life experience, attitude, beliefs and body state are crucial to our interventions. Our orientation and experiences in dance and movement will affect the programme we create with our groups, as will our relationships with ourselves, and with the group and movement processes. Our own dance is the wellspring of inspiration and, as such, needs cherishing.

Note

1 The term dance/movement therapy is used in the USA, whereas in most European and other countries around the world it is written as 'dance therapy' or 'dance movement therapy'. In the UK the term now employed is 'dance movement psychotherapy'.

PRACTICAL AND THEORETICAL ISSUES

Developmental movement processes

An understanding of developmental movement can help to give the leader a starting-point for some activities, especially with those groups that have a developmental lag. A developmental movement structure (see pp. 39–47) may be given in one session or divided and presented sequentially over several sessions. The whole structure may be used on specific stages only. The following is a brief overview of the motoric development that normally takes place in early childhood. Structures that may be used to illuminate and re-create these stages are then built around the process.

Motor patterns

Some people may have criticisms of the stages presented, based upon their own experience; however, the patterns shown are those that can generally be expected in normal development. A developing infant may omit some stages altogether, whilst others may need to be consolidated longer. In normal development one thing is certain: physical growth will always take place with accompanying motor patterns. None the less environment and physical opportunity can affect these patterns.

A knowledge of these patterns can enable any practitioner to provide for consolidation and/or the next stage in motor development, for example with clients who have a developmental lag, or to encourage clients' re-experiencing of specific stages. By referring to the figures you can follow the summary of the motoric stages of development at monthly frequencies. It is important to note that some of the motoric embodiments may trigger emotional material for some participants.

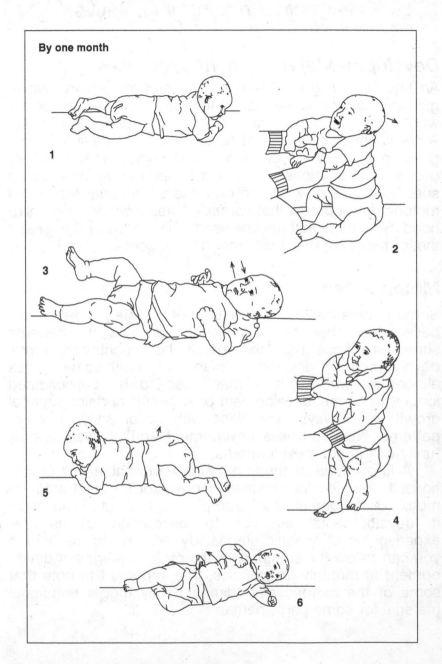

By one month

1

2

3

4

5

6

By one month

At birth the infant can turn its head, focus on objects and usually has flexed limbs, with hands near to the face. It has a strong sucking action, roots for the nipple and shows a grasp in its hands by which it can be lifted. The startle reflex, where both arms shoot outwards if it is shocked or roughly handled, is prevalent, later to be lost, as is the rigid body position when held horizontally.

Drawing 1 shows the infant on its front; it can raise its head slightly.

Drawing 2 shows the infant being held sitting; its head falls backwards.

Drawing 3 shows the infant flexing and extending arms and legs and turning its head from side to side while on its back.

Drawing 4 shows the walking reflex action, which is lost soon after birth. The infant will flex and extend its knees alternately when held upright with the sole of the foot on a surface.

Drawing 5 shows the infant raising its pelvis and flexing its knees to make a crawling action, although there is no forward movement as yet.

Drawing 6 shows the infant rolling from its side onto its back, often with the heavy head leading and the back arching.

By two months

Drawing 1 shows the infant on its front, raising its head to 45 degrees and its torso onto its forearms.

Drawing 2 shows the infant being held in a sitting position, where its head wobbles and its back is weak.

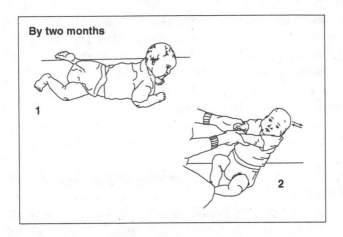

By two months

By three months

Drawing 1 shows the infant finding and exploring its hands; it is also noticing and touching other body parts, such as its feet. It can involuntarily grasp objects on contact and raises its head forward when held sitting.

Drawing 2 shows the infant's hips extended while it is lying on its back.

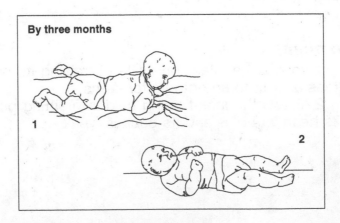

By three months

By four months

Drawing 1 shows that the infant can now raise its upper torso onto its elbows and lift its head to 90 degrees.

Drawing 2 shows the infant rolling from its back onto its side; it can now hold its back upright when sitting, but it is still weak. It can hold its head up unaided.

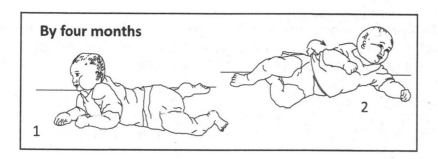

By four months

By five months

Drawing 1 shows the infant with its hands flat open on the floor as it raises its upper torso, pushing strongly away from the floor. At this stage its grasp is voluntary, and it actively aims to reach objects.

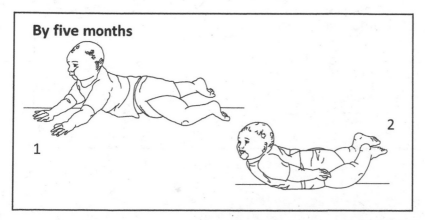

By five months

Drawing 2 shows the infant supporting itself on its thorax. At this stage it can actively help in postures such as sitting and extends and flexes all its limbs while exploring body parts (touching its feet, for example).

By six months

Drawing 1 shows the infant raised up on its open hands when in the prone position. The head is back, and the neck strongly supports it.

Drawing 2 shows the infant lifting its head up and forward when lying on its back, abdominal muscles becoming stronger. At this stage the infant can stand with help (often on tips of toes).

Drawing 3 shows the infant picking up objects with one hand while supporting itself with the other, when prone.

Drawing 4 shows the infant rolling from front to back.

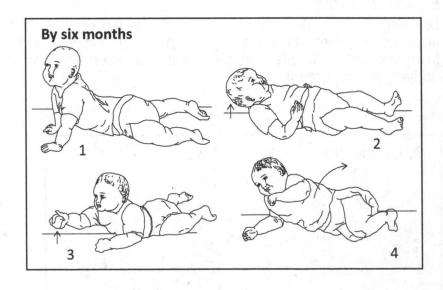

By six months

By seven months

Drawing 1 shows the infant sitting upright without support; hands are often forward on the floor to prevent falling.
Drawing 2 shows the infant rolling from its back to its front. Often rocking movements initiate this stage.
Drawing 3 shows the 'letting go' of objects.

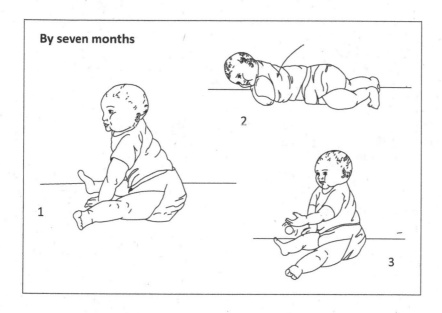

By seven months

By eight months

Drawing 1 shows that the infant can sit alone and has good muscle tones.
Drawing 2 shows the infant rolling in both directions.
Drawing 3 shows the infant rolling itself from lying to sitting.
Drawing 4 shows the infant raising itself from prone to bearing weight on hands and toes. By this stage it may have pushed itself along on its back with its feet, moved around in a circle on its front/back and made swimming/pushing actions while prone.

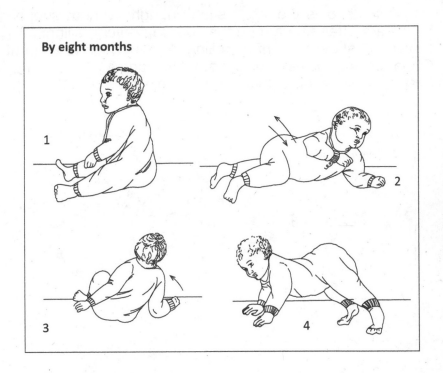

By eight months

By nine months

Drawing 1 shows the infant rocking back and forth to begin crawling, often backwards at first.

Drawing 2 shows that the infant needs to hold on to furniture/people to balance in the upright position (hips out behind). Falling occurs frequently at this stage.

By eleven months

Drawing 1 shows that the child can walk while supporting itself on a wide base.

Drawing 2 shows that the child can 'bear walk' on alternate limbs, 'all fours'.

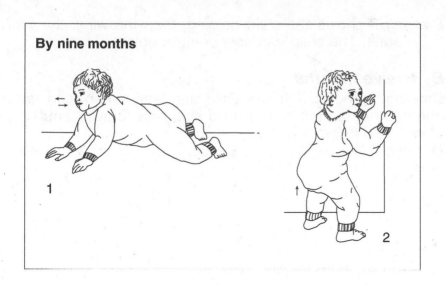

By nine months

1

2

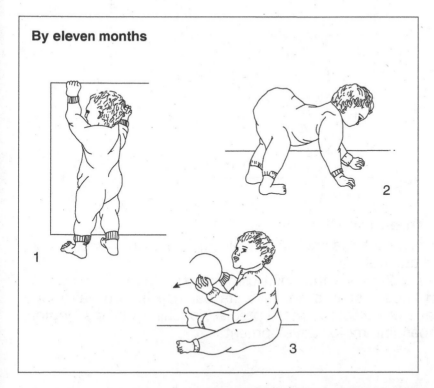

By eleven months

1

2

3

Drawing 3 shows the child holding, then throwing, the ball to an adult. The child can now point at objects.

By twelve months

Drawing 1 shows that the child can walk when held with one hand by an adult. The child sits, rolls, crawls, shuffles, stands and falls.

Drawing 2 shows the child bending to pick up a released object.

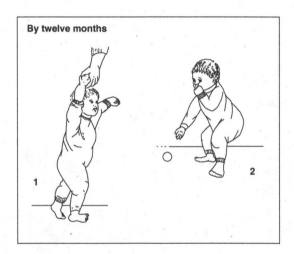

By fifteen months

Drawing 1 shows the child walking alone on a wide base, arms outstretched.

Drawing 2 shows the child climbing stairs on all fours. The child kneels, stands up, falls. Its balance is poor, although release of objects is more precise; pushing objects begins, as does fine motor development.

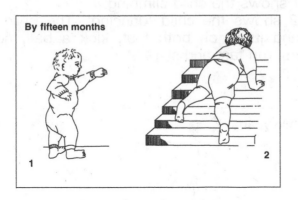

By fifteen months

By eighteen months

Drawing 1 shows the child climbing stairs with an adult.
Drawing 2 shows the child running with a wide base; falls may occur. It can jump with feet together, pull a toy behind, walk backwards, and push a ball with its feet.

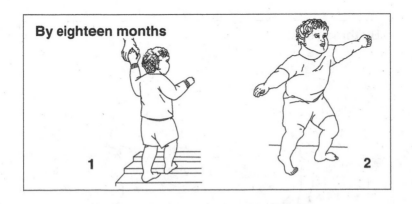

By eighteen months

By two years

Drawing 1 shows the child climbing.
Drawing 2 shows the child 'dancing'. The child can now balance and jump on both feet, kick a ball, go up and down stairs, run fast and skip.

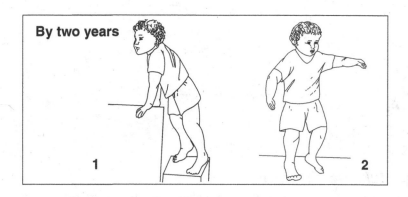

By three years

Drawing 1 shows the child jumping on one foot (hop). Balance is now good; it leaps, hops; alternate arms swing in walk.
Drawing 2 shows the young child riding a tricycle.

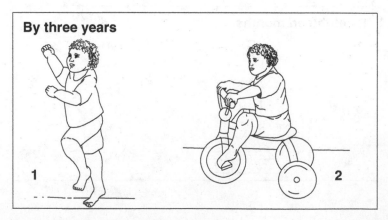

Possible developmental movement structures

These structures can be employed whatever the intention and anticipated outcomes. A possible developmental movement structure demonstrated in structure A below could be employed within a DMP session. There may be specific aims/objectives to be considered concerning the group, and its needs to pay attention to, as well as safe practice.

In the suggested structure B below, when offered by the dance and movement practitioner it will be more of a straightforward physical experience, perhaps to foster a greater sequencing of the developmental stages and recapitulate any motor patterns that perhaps have been missed or have yet to be reached by the individual. It can become a sort of rehabilitative exercise for some populations.

Use language that will be appropriate for your client group. Please note that this is not designed as a rebirthing experience (see Glossary); an in-depth training is required for this (see Section 4). Feel free to use your own words once you have a sense of the structure.

Possible developmental movement structure A

Lead the group through the structure by saying something like the following:

1 'Become aware of the space in the room, then find a place on the floor you feel comfortable in. Find a way to get down to the floor, then close your eyes.'
2 'Find a comfortable curled position. Imagine you are in a perfect environment. You have no needs, and all flows in your movement; your exploration of hands, toes, body is accidental. You turn over, stretch and bend. You are in the womb, getting ready to be born.'
3 'This is birth—the first pain in life. You are moving forward and being moved towards a new environment.

Your eyes open wide to find that it is bright and noisy, the air is cold, and you cry and breathe alone for the first time. You hear your own sound and your mother's sound in a different way. You rest, very tired.'

(Do not spend long in this phase; the purpose of this structure is to experience a range of movements as if for the first time, not to re-live the birth itself.)

4 'Your hands, closed or open, often go to your mouth. You start to make other very small movements, unable to do much. Different body parts move—your back, elbows, knees, hands and feet. You move onto your stomach and feel your contact with the floor. You move your arms and chest and find that you can push up and away from the floor. You can rock from side to side and forward and back. These are your first attempts at loco-motion [see Glossary]. Your eyes may be open or closed; whenever they open you look up and out. You can now support your weight with your hands. You kick strongly.'

5 'Now you can hold your head up, with the neck muscles much stronger. You experience being upright in this sense. Roll from side to side; this is your first large movement. Now you can start to crawl to get around, and you move to grasp things that attract you. You can change your own environment by locomotion. Can you remember the kind of house you were in when you first crawled? Who was there? You can change from crawling to sitting upright to kneeling to shifting forward on your seat. You use forward, sideways and backwards directions.'

6 'Now you can stand while holding onto something, your feet wide apart and very unsteady. Being vertical is a new dimension. Someone helps you walk forward. You test out your mobility and stumble or fall but are excited at the freedom of movement as you move alone for the first time.'

7 'You can now succeed and fail at those first steps. Step, step quickly and grab hold, totter, fall. You choose where to go, explore the environment. Step onto, pull onto, pull through and reach over objects. You practice your walk.'

8 'Now as you get older and more confident your walk becomes a run, then, later, a jump with both feet; then continue leaping, hopping, doing somersaults and balances, climbing and skipping. Where are you: at school, with brothers or sisters?'

9 'Notice others but play alongside rather than with them. Perhaps follow or copy a movement. Touch and interact. Test your new-found movements against other people's. Try not to talk. Groups form spontaneously— join and leave them, choosing to remain or ignore them and be alone. Where are you at this stage? Can you remember a particular place?'

10 'Now you are 11 to 12 years old, independent yet dependent. You like cuddles still. Your body is beginning to change, and you are aware of how you appear to others. How are you moving?'

11 'You are 14 to 16 years old now, frustrated, angry and bored. Who are you? There are big questions in life. Friends and looking alike are very important to you. Your sexual identity is developing. You are neither an adult nor a child. How do you move? What kind of walk do you have? What kind of rhythm does it have?'

12 'You are 16 to 18 years old now, struggling with decisions about boy/girlfriends, perhaps your first car and job. You form close friendships; you may feel conflict and rebellion.'

13 'At 20 to 30 years you feel safer as you grow and mature. Find your own movement signature—how do you move now? With what preferences? Slowly, quickly, strongly, softly? Lots of factors in your life make up your movement style. Is it work, people, sports, nurturing roles? Allow movement to happen; this could have a repetitive pattern that is like a metaphor

for your life. What sound or word or image accompanies it? What colour is it?'

14 'As you get older your rhythm changes; how does the movement change? What are the limitations? Any sound, images? Bones are more fragile, it's not so easy to get up, sit down or find a resting place. You feel satisfied, relaxed. Breathing is easy. Reflect on your life.'

15 Group feedback.

Possible developmental movement structure B

1 'Lie on your back in a space as though you were a young infant.'
2 'Open out while lying on your back and make opening and closing movements with your limbs.'
3 'Explore your toes and fingers; grasp and release.'
4 'Roll over onto your front, allowing the head to lead. Lift the head, push up your chest and rock forward and back.'
5 'Pull yourself along, pushing with knees and feet. Push yourself along on your back, using both your feet.'
6 'Crawl, creep, sit up, turn and lie down. Repeat this sequence of movements so that they flow one after the other.'
7 'Bottom shuffle along, fall forward, backward and sideways, catching yourself with your hands. Change direction of locomotion.'
8 'Do "bear walks" (on all fours, feet and hands in contact with the ground, arms and legs extended).'
9 'Stand up, holding onto a stable object; fall down, fight gravity again, raise your hips and let your weight fall onto your legs.'
10 'Climb onto objects, then stand alone as if for the first time.'
11 'Take a few first steps alone.'
12 'Walk, run, walk, climb and run.'
13 'Leap, first from one foot then from both.'
14 'Jump with feet together, hop, balance and skip.'

15 'Repeat the above but with a partner assisting the movement experiences, for example helping rolls, standing and catching. The partner makes contact with your head (e.g. by resting a hand upon it lightly) to ensure that it leads the movement. The partner helps in forward, backward, and stretched and curled sideways rolls. For example, support their forward roll by having them roll over your shoulder while you are sitting with legs astride. Help them to curl over and around their centre while you maintain contact with hands on their head and body.'

Non-verbal communication as expression and communication within the group

Movement, as a medium for dance, is the expressive and communicative aspect of human development. Espenak (1981) elaborates:

> By the term dance we can refer to an entire constellation of physical expression. In so far as movement, gesture or posture, represents communication to the self, leader or group—that movement is dance.
>
> (p. 2)

Movement is at the core of our development and has a profound influence on the learning of speech, socially acceptable behaviour and cognitive skills. In this sense we are looking, not at functional movement—that is, movement in which a skill is performed as in specific dance techniques, sports or lifting a cup to drink—but at the expressive movement form. Extensive research has been carried out on the observation of movement and its emotional communication; see, for example, Birdwhistell (1970), Condon (1969), Lamb (1979), North (1972) and Hall (1973). It is this observable relationship between emotion and motion that is expressive of the individual. Body posture, facial grimaces, the strength of a handshake and other movements found in social communication have much in common with creative dance.

Amongst the basic assumptions of using creative dance and movement processes as vehicles for change is that, by changing the body so that it functions differently in movement terms, we promote a corresponding effect on the mind when both are focused on together. Trudi Schoop (1973), a well-known early pioneer in dance therapy from California, wrote:

> If I am correct in assuming mind and body are interactive, I feel a problem of disturbance can be influenced from either side. When psychoanalysis brings about a change in the mental attitude there should be a corresponding change in body behaviour. And when dance therapy brings about a change in the body there should be a corresponding change in the mind. The approach to verbal psychotherapy is through the mind–body and the approach to dance therapy is through the body—mind. Both methods want to change the whole being.
>
> (p. 45)

However, we must be cautious about taking for granted a simple mind–body equation, that is assuming that what happens physically happens in an equivalent way in the structure of the human psyche. A person is their body, not the possessor of their body. To change the mind—body is to change the shape of the self. People need to deal adequately with the changing shapes of their lives, a process of continual reorganisation, which Piaget (1952) called 'accommodation'. Habitual patterns of movement, frequently based on early pre-verbal experiences, are often the only resource we have to make sense of the world. When we become stuck in those patterns, as in reactive behaviour, learning new behaviours is imperative if we are to grow and integrate changes. When initiating creative action in movement another resource for dealing with life changes is made available. Some patterns we have are no longer relevant to our healthy functioning and need to adapt to our present needs.

The advantage of focusing on the movement behaviour is that the body is often more pliable, plastic and capable of reorganisation than is our thinking. The body does not lie about itself, but we can lie about the body. The body is capable of regenerating, reshaping itself and growing. Changes on a biochemical and neuromuscular level can be initiated by the person themselves; this is the basis of bio-feedback techniques.

To alter a life situation is to change not just through the mind alone but through the way the self is used. A change in the body's behaviour can often be facilitated by non-verbal means at a primary level of functioning, that is, at the felt level (Gendlin, 1962), allowing an expression of repressed and important emotions. The movement phases alone, as in going through the motions, are not enough in themselves: the emotional aspects must be worked with in conjunction with the physical. Clients who resist movement need to be helped gradually to initiate their own involve-ment. 'Not moving' or 'stillness' is equally important; it is not necessary to be engaged in gross bodily movement to participate. By observing the subtle, shadowy movements an involvement may result. However small the steps, the leader needs to be sensitive to the way this involvement is developed. The leader's movement range is the resource that enables the participant to move in less accessible dir-ections, levels, dimensions and combinations of qualities, creating and exploring other forms of expression.

Developing creative dance as expression and communication within the group

The raw materials for dance are rhythm and pattern. As dis-cussed above, one could say that any movement is dance—look at slowed down or speeded up film or video-tape; a pattern of rhythmical spatial structures can be seen.

Stern (1979) refers to the choreography between the mother and child.

Movement can be classified into three types: functional or instrumental (as in, for example, picking up a cup to drink, akin to Allport's (1961) coping behaviour); quantitative (as in, for example, running fast in sport); and qualitative (as in the expression of moods and feelings and in expressive and aesthetic qualities). Sandle (1975) has discussed these at some length. It is the last type with which we are concerned here, that of the qualitative dynamics of movement.

To find a movement is success enough for some clients; making it into a dance may be too difficult because of their level of functioning. Thus we need to work developmentally, going from simple movement play and developmental processes (see pp. 39–43) towards symbolic movement and communicative dance. When developing the group's movement, it may be possible for them to improvise, then select and link movements together. Once the selection process is complete the client may be able to organise and pattern the movements and to make transitions between selected movements.

When mastery such as this is attained, the client will have a movement vocabulary in which to acknowledge, express and communicate within the group, sometimes sharing their dance with the group. Learning the language is part of the process, as in verbal psychotherapy. The dance needs to be repeated and rehearsed to develop or provoke any movement memory. This repetition is a means of exploration and of establishing a personal reality.

Carl Rogers (1967), one of America's most distinguished psychologists, said:

> Learning itself is dependent on wanting to learn, it depends on not knowing the answers but on being willing to explore. It is idiosyncratic and can only significantly influence behaviour if it is self-appropriated learning; truth that has been assimilated in experience.

Movement is experience, and, as with learning, engagement with it is dependent on a willingness to move. Self-understanding is the process of an unfolding adventure common to all learning. As the dance flows into the regressive and out again it offers the freedom for new growth, to rediscover developmental patterns and personal significance in birth, lying, rolling, rocking, kneeling, crawling, standing and walking (see pp. 27–39).

In dance the body is able to re-experience as the sensor, medium and actor, receiving and responding to kinaesthetic, rhythmical and social stimuli. The client becomes aware of their body and its parts, of the numerous possibilities for moving in time and space with varying amounts of energy and effort, and of moving with their own unique patterns. The process of moving is rewarding for its own sake; Schilder (1950) described it as 'loosening up one's body image'.

Structured movement activities based on the client's own repertoire can lead to improvisation on themes as they emerge. Confidence is gained when movement is repeated and takes place in different contexts, as with a partner or an object. Eventually the client internalises the feeling in the dance and this may become registered at an unconscious level. By making subtle changes in the expressive movement as the group moves together in a group improvisation, the leader reflects the group, yet provides alternatives that may or may not be mirrored by the group.

The process is designed to take the group on a journey from where they are to an extension of that 'here and now'. For example, the movement perseveration (see Glossary) of 'rocking', often seen in populations labelled 'autistic' or with severe learning difficulties, may be rediscovered together on the floor, standing or with one person supporting the other. Arms or whole bodies may be rocked, side to side or forward and back. Here the movement is focused upon, although vocalisation and expressive language play an important role with groups who have these possibilities, as does insight. During a mirroring dance in a group or with an individual in the group the leader can gradually make changes in the timing, use of space or effort (see 'Laban movement analysis' below) and say any words that may express the feeling sense of the movement; some clients, equally, may verbalise or make sounds. This extends repertoire for 'shaping' and 'effort' responses, allowing a wider range of experience in the emotional counterpart to the movement.

The starting-point may come from a theme that developed from a previous session, such as saying goodbye, or it may be something going on at present for the group or individual. It may be exploring a movement theme such as 'opening' or 'closing', or 'jumping'.

A jumping dance might begin with lots of different kinds of jumps. The group can be guided to improvise, then select some favourites or non-favourites to organise and master. Their choice may reflect their mood, their range may be extensive or restrictive; however, it cannot be wrong. To encourage expansion in movement, alternatives are to increase the ability to express moods, attitudes, ideas and behaviours. The jumping dance, once mastered and remembered, may begin to evoke images. These could be explored: for example, fear of falling or always wanting to be up in the sky and never being happy in contact with the ground. Where possible, discussion then makes connections, after which it is important to go back to the movement experience and reshape it with new consciousness.

It is only when the emotional is worked with in parallel to the physical that change in attitude, self-image and understanding can come about and growth towards full potential can begin. This is the difference between teaching dance, and dance movement psychotherapy; the contract is different. Motion and emotion are inextricably intertwined. Movement may be emotionally motivated. The emotion and its intensity evoke the movement; for example, we lunge into assertiveness, squeeze ourselves with delight, stand on our own feet. We are how we move. It is when this is brought into consciousness that changes can take place. The rhythmic nature of dance can bring organisation to what may be a disordered and confused individual or group. Patterns and sequencing of movement and its repetition can help to give the internal locus of control needed by those who are 'acting out'. In addition, non-verbal signals may be more accurately responded to if the client has first been sensitised to their own non-verbal communication and that of others in sessions.

The movement processes themselves are expressive statements in the group, for example, where people place themselves in space in relation to each other and the leader.

In conclusion, however complex the psychopathology of the clients, communication through movement can touch them. We have the same inherent needs and barriers to communication, trust and relationship often found in people with mental health needs or disabilities. These barriers can be seen in their body boundaries (see Glossary), body image, use of space and movement. They can be overcome by working with their conflicts and motivating their desire for contact and growth, thereby giving them opportunities to form constructive relationships. The pre-verbal, felt and symbolic nature of movement and dance can enable feelings to be identified, explored and expressed, the body, feelings and mind acting as one during the movement.

Work at a verbal and non-verbal level can allow for the felt level to be transformed into body movement through imagery. In those who are able, this precipitates verbal expression at the appropriate developmental level. The reliance on spontaneity and creativity gives a chance for self-directed behaviour and choices and helps release 'frozen', confining behavioural responses and habitual effort patterns (many clients manifest excessive use of one or more of the motion factors, as in, for example, hyperactivity or flaccidity). However, it may be necessary to focus on helping the group learn to feel confident in their own spontaneity; or to emphasise learning to play. These new, alternative movement patterns built into the movement vocabulary, with corresponding work with the psychophysical state, can provide the choice of recovery of experiences and can act as a balancing factor for a wider response to the environment.

It is important for anyone using dance movement as a vehicle for growth to be aware of their own movement habits, preferences and psychophysical states in addition to having at their disposal a wide movement repertoire to create a non-verbal rapport with the group, using varying qualities, tensions, speeds and so on, enabling other forms of expression and ways of being to emerge.

Effective sessions will depend upon many factors, but specifically upon training and experience in the field of non-stylised dance, group process psychotherapy and a dance movement psychotherapy training (see 'Training in dance movement psychotherapy', pp. 337–342).

Planning and evaluating a programme

Achievement of physical and emotional integration allows an individual to be more responsive to the environment. Dance and movement activities in a planned programme can help to optimise this integration by:

1 providing for growth in individual identity; affirmation and the emergence of self through the formation of an adequate body image;
2 improving social capabilities; developing contact, trust, sensitivity and co-operation with others to enhance decision-making skills and self-confidence;
3 giving opportunities for expressive use of the body, drawing upon emotional and imaginative resources;
4 giving a sense of achievement;
5 generalising movement patterns into a wider variety of situations;

6 improving functional and dynamic elements of a skill, such as neuromuscular skills in co-ordination of walking;

7 providing the range of movement needed to allow choice in organising, interpreting and manipulating the world.

Activities involved in your session may or may not be accompanied by music (see 'The use of music', pp. 337–342). Where music is used you will need to be aware of the 'feeling component' of it. Use it to reflect or contrast with the group feeling. Participants may choose the music or bring in their favourite Spotify playlist/CDs. These can often act as motivation in the warm-up.

Goals for sessions may be set by the group as a whole, individuals, the staff, the leader or a combination of all these. Goals may be to do with where to go in the group's explorations; group members may even specify the particular behaviour they wish to change, although this does not mean that they are necessarily willing to engage with that change. The 'moving experience' itself may help to uncover goals as well as the realisation of goals. It is important to help clients reflect on their own experience of the session and to aim at small steps, rather than letting them think the sessions will make everything in their lives wonderful. For some groups a pre-treatment interview may be helpful in clarifying what sessions are about and what they feel they could gain. For other groups such an interview may only heighten anxiety levels.

Discussion, feedback and self-disclosure may follow an activity and often connections are made by participants about their experience and realities. It is useful to return again to the movement form, repeating it with this more conscious awareness, noticing what might change and facilitating experimentation with other ways of being.

All sessions need careful thought, and after each session it is crucial to spend time on evaluation, both as a reflection on that session and as a preparation for the planning of the succeeding session.

The development of a session can be seen as a 'creative energy cycle', moving on from the nurturing in the warm-up, to energising in the introduction of the theme, to the climax where the theme is developed in the middle of the session, through to closure where a warm-down finishes the session.

Each stage of the session will vary in length, depending on the phase of development of the group. Warm-ups are generally longer in the early sessions than later on in the group life, but in any event normally do not last more than one-quarter of the total session time. Similarly, the warm-down stage should not last more than the final quarter of the session; group members here should be encouraged to leave as individuals separating from the group.

The main work takes place in the middle of the session, where the leader will have selected activities that will help to develop the group themes. These middle stages should take up about half the session time. Introduction of the theme focuses the attention and the development stage involves participants in deeper stimulation.

Ideally the energy cycle should appear as shown in Figure 2.1. This indicates that the group begins and ends with a lower energy level than that found in the middle of a session. Relaxation activities, reflection through verbalisation, integration processes, and awareness focusing on everyday things outside the group can help the transition to closure. You need to ensure that the warm-down finishes in time to close the session punctually. You may need to warn the group that there are only 10, then 5, then 2 minutes left. Always time the activities and let the group know how much time they have at the beginning and have left at the end of each activity.

From the previous session's evaluation, it will be evident that a theme has evolved that can be developed in the succeeding session. After deciding upon the overall framework, specific activities that facilitate work on that

Figure 2.1 **The creative energy cycle**

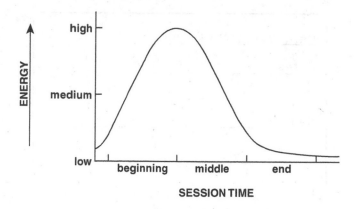

theme can be planned. However, be prepared for another theme to emerge from the group's warm-up. This may be more relevant to work with at that stage. The leader may choose to reflect the theme or work with its opposite. The linking of themes from session to session gives continuity to the group. In a short time the group will have a life of its own, where particular themes emerging can be selected by the leader as being suitable to work with, given the length of time the group will be together, and the members' life situations, functioning and anxiety levels. The group responds to the structure provided in a spontaneous, organic manner. The leader will be able to change the structure and activities according to their moods and needs to maintain this spontaneity.

You may find it appropriate, when collecting referrals for your group, to interview each potential participant individually. You may find it helps them to understand the aims and context of the anticipated group and thus be in a position to volunteer to become a participant. Asking them about their expectations of such a group and of movement might also be helpful. Sometimes a written contract can be designed (see Figure 2.2 for an example) and

Practical and theoretical issues 53

Figure 2.2 **Example of a contract for ground rules**

```
Re :   Movement Group ____

Dates : _____


Name : _____

Date : _____

I _____ agree to
participate in the group
described to me. I understand
that total confidentiality
will be respected and that
my contribution will be used
entirely for the group's purposes.




Signature : _____
```

signed by the members. Demonstration sessions are another important aspect of giving an idea to possible participants of what the sessions will be about. Ensure a range of activities are provided for the demonstration session. Expectations need to be verbalised, both from the practitioner/therapist and from the group to the practitioner/therapist.

The first session establishes the initial working relationship with the group as a whole. For those groups with expressive and receptive language abilities, ground rules and the general purpose of the group can be discussed and agreed upon together. This can help engender co-operation and self-responsibility in the group. The ground rules and aims of the group will need to be reviewed regularly and possibly amended. The group and practitioner/therapist need to be clear as to what happens if ground rules are broken. Maintenance of boundaries is essential to promote group cohesion and a culture of trust. Any contract needs to reflect the intention of the group, whether therapy or a movement/dance group. For the latter there may not be a need to limit confidentiality and/or instigate confidentiality as a ground rule.

Confidentiality

The European Union General Data Protection Regulation (GDPR) (www.EUGDPR.org.uk) is relevant for all sectors to any professional holding sensitive and detailed personal information on clients. It is important to be aware of compliance duties, as it does affect practice and systems as appropriate to the contractual arrangements in the setting. Check where responsibility lies for leading on or contributing to data renewal, whether self-employed, working privately, or contracted in an organisation, to ensure you are working within the law. GDPR sets a high standard for consent, aiming to build a culture of transparency to enable clients to make informed choices. You may need to review what this means for your consent procedures. Data storage processes, for example, need to be 'live' and must be reviewed at least every six months. Consent should be unambiguous and a clear, affirmative action, separate from any other terms and conditions, not a precondition of signing up for a service. Pre-ticked boxes are banned, records to demonstrate consent must be kept, and clients must be informed that they can withdraw consent at any time without negative consequences. If clients' data are to be used for writing, research or training, consent should include a list stating how data will be presented, who will have access to it, how it will be published and any consequences of public publishing. Clients should be requested to give consent to each usage individually rather than a blanket consent. Include a statement confirming that clients' responses regarding data usage will not affect their right to access therapy or classes. When working with children and young people for whom gaining parental/carer/guardian consent may be required, in exceptional circumstances be aware of the Gillick competency law and Fraser guidelines. Volunteers and trainees are no different to employees in that they must undergo training. You must be trained and equipped to protect data. The training on placement involves the trainee holding responsibility for ensuring they manage the risks adequately. If you are self-employed you need to register with the ICO as data controllers and data processors as the GDPR places specific responsibilities on you such as maintaining records of personal data and processing activities, with a legal liability if there is a breach. It is suggested that only clinical notes are kept, and process recordings are shredded as soon as appropriate.

For a therapy group, however, the limits of confidentiality need articulating clearly to members, such as the limits (i.e. if you suspect there is, or may be, any possible harm to themselves or others) for safeguarding procedures. There will also need to be clarification that certain aspects of the groupwork will be discussed with a supervisor in confidence, and possibly extended to any multi-disciplinary team at case conferences, for example.

Ground rules

The contract example of suggested ground rules below (Figure 2.2) may be amended to suit either type of group.

The following ground rules have been used in practice (these do not need to be in a written form), however all group members need to agree to adhere to them prior to the commencement of the group whatever the intention/context. For some groups the ground rules can be decided upon together to encourage ownership:

1 The session will begin and end on time. All members are responsible for ensuring this happens (the practitioner/therapist gives times of sessions and number of sessions for which the group will meet; any breaks, such as holidays or employment of locums need to be clarified here).
2 No physical damage to self, others or the environment is permitted (some jewelry might need to be removed).
3 Confidentiality: (Clarify this with GDPR in mind. Giving a handout on GDPR might be useful for some groups). The content of the group will not be disclosed outside the session unless specifically agreed with the group or individual beforehand (bearing in mind limits to confidentiality as appropriate).
4 Each member is responsible for their own participation, although you will encourage all to become involved.
5 No smoking, drinking, eating or chewing gum during the session.
6 Participants are encouraged to stay in the space during the session, or if required, they can request a short 3-minute comfort break.

The ground rules, levels of discussion about them and any contract will all depend on the setting, the purpose of the group and the clients' level of functioning. You will need to clarify participants' personal aims for the group as well as any professional aims you will have. In a team situation, integration of aims already set for clients will need to be incorporated.

It is a good idea to develop a ritual (see Glossary) at the start of the session early in the group life; this may be anything from 'participants removing their shoes' to something more complex that evolves from the group material. Whatever it is, it needs to relax the group and promote anticipation of the session. Rituals to close sessions are sometimes appropriate too. Rituals can be included in the ground rules; they provide safety and help in developing group cohesion.

Setting the climate and creating group cohesion and promoting alliance

It is essential that groups feel safe for any change to take place. Creating a safe environment and facilitating interactive activities early in the session, therefore, can prepare the group to engage in later, more in-depth work. These preparatory practices can help to set the climate for the subsequent sessions.

Group climate is a significant factor concerning how interactions between participants and a leader affect the atmosphere in the group (Choi, Price and Vinokur, 2003). The climate may determine participants' ability and motivation to express feelings, thoughts, ideas and beliefs, thus their engagement with the group (Harel, Shechtman and Cutrona, 2011). Open communication and trusting relationships between participants make up a supportive group climate. Specific practices at the beginning of an intervention/programme engage participants in developing trust between each other and with the practitioner/leader/therapist to encourage a beneficial atmosphere. Participants' perception of the climate can affect interactions, however, since perception can reflect individual representations of the group based on prior experience of groups (e.g. the family). A positive perception of the group climate may indicate a view that the group is trustworthy and therefore safe to explore and practice new skills. Kivlighan and Tarrant (2001) concur, suggesting that when participants are active and engaged this is related to viewing the group as beneficial, supported by Ogrodniczuk and Piper (2003) who showed a correlation between group climate and therapeutic gain, whether positive or negative, depending on the level of conflict and the stage of the development. Furthermore, in an active, experiential group, preparing participants for the subsequent planned activities at the start of sessions is helpful in developing the group. For example, individual breath and vocal work might be undertaken at the start if individual moving with the breath and vocalising are to be worked with in the middle stage of the session. Alternatively, if quiet introspection is required for some later partner work, then the warm-up could reflect a quiet atmosphere, with group members perhaps mindfully breathing as they walk in pairs, side by side, around and through the space.

Group cohesion and interpersonal learning, according to Yalom and Leszcz (2005), are important to capture group themes in relation to individual themes. They propose that by understanding and examining the group's interaction and its effects on the process, the individual and the group will be helped. The group that examines itself originated as the T-group (Rogers, 1970), a humanistic person-centred approach. Yalom and Leszcz (2005) emphasised the attribution of interpersonal relationships and cognitive understanding to the meaning of the process.

Group cohesion describes the relationship quality with other participants and the group's and participants' perception of the leader/therapist/practitioner as, for example, being genuine, competent, warm. Cohesiveness is therefore a significant factor in groupwork. This feeling of 'togetherness' creates a safe environment whilst at the same time enabling a group's active engagement with self-disclosure, challenge and interpersonal conflict. Yalom and Leszcz (2005) claim cohesiveness is a strong determinant of positive therapeutic outcomes, when outcome is defined as reducing symptom distress or improvement in interpersonal functioning. Studies such as Budman et al. (1989) evaluated cohesiveness in different settings and modalities (such as in-patient, experiential/gestalt) and found it significantly determines outcomes such as improved self-esteem and reduction of symptoms

Cohesion does not signify 'groupthink' (Janis, 1982) characterised by the pressure to conform and maintain consensus under all circumstances. In contrast, whilst it promotes a sense of belonging, group cohesiveness in psychotherapy also demands critical thinking on the part of the individual members (Yalom and Leszcz, 2005).

Promoting group cohesiveness is not only essential in the context of psychotherapy. Cohesion refers to the quality of relationships that develop between participants and the practitioner/facilitator/therapist/leader/educator so will be central to any successful groupwork and it is advisable to emphasise interaction between all.

The facilitation of group cohesion is critical to the appeal the group has for participants, and to their sense of safety and belonging in the group. Group cohesion can be defined as 'the result of all the forces acting on all the members such that they remain in the group, or, more simply, the attractiveness of the group to its members' (Yalom and Leszcz, 2005, p. 55). Therefore, group cohesion is vital for ensuring people do not withdraw from the group, which jeopardises safety. MacKenzie (1997) proposes group cohesion is a general term for the quality of the whole group based on group integration and individual attraction to the group. Consequently, empathy, emotional connection and attraction once established can result in a greater willingness to self-disclose, feelings of trust, respect, acceptance, safety, comfort and caring. It can also refer to what extent participants have a shared goal, feel part of something, valued, supported by others and are committed to the goals and task of the group (Dinger and Schauenburg, 2010; Harel, Shechtman and Cutrona, 2011).

Risk-taking in giving feedback and establishing interpersonal relationships is more possible in a cohesive group (Yalom and Leszcz, 2005). Furthermore, participation increases, producing more interactions, leading to a more productive, effective group with improved outcomes in an upward spiral (Johnson and Johnson, 2013).

Hornsey, Dwyer and Oei (2007) showed that strong identification with a group connects to greater commitment, loyalty and trust, creating a positive outcome for the group, as did Burlingame, Fuhriman and Johnson (2002, 2004; Burlingame, McClendon and Alonso, 2011). Burlingame et al. identified specific group behaviours: self-disclosure, feedback, group leader and participants' contributions, and increased cohesion. Cohesion is associated with the stage of the group and develops over time. The more developed the group, usually the more cohesive it is. There is evidence that a group lasting more than 12 sessions, composed of between five and nine participants, has greater cohesion (Burlingame, McClendon and Alonso, 2011). Younger participants experience the largest outcome changes when cohesion is present within their groups. Fostering cohesion will be particularly useful for those working in college counselling centres and with adolescent populations (ibid). Group cohesion strengthens after periods of stress/conflict whereby group and personal issues that need time for participants to feel safe enough to process are addressed and resolved (Yalom and Leszcz, 2005), thus cohesion tends to rely on the timeframe of the group.

Early cohesion can lead to increased productivity and positive outcomes. Participants are already in a state of commitment to the group's aim and thus willing to work and explore relationships and personal issues (Corey, 2012). Cohesion is more important to establish early on in short-term groups with less time to develop a sense of safety (Marmarosh and Van Horn, 2010).

Group climate and cohesion are traditionally associated with whole groupwork phenomena, whereas the notions of alliance and empathy originated in individual therapy. Group alliance is an important factor referring to the therapeutic relationship between participants and the practitioner/therapist/leader, based on 'here and now' encounters (Horvath, 2006). Group climate, cohesion and alliance indicate differences in relationships relative to group content, roles taken up (member to member, member to leader and member to group) and the quality of those relationships (Bakali, Baldwin and Lorentzen, 2009). Research indicates that each of these factors are highly related to one another, serve similar functions and can give indications of outcomes (Johnson et al., 2005, 2006).

A bi-directional relationship exists between the group process at various stages and the way it deals with issues; the stage can signify the group content and vice versa. The stage is linked to the development of cohesion, group climate and alliance. For example, Tuckman (1965) outlined a linear four-stage model of group development: forming, storming, norming and performing. Tuckman and Jensen (2010) later added a fifth stage, adjourning. MacKenzie and Livesley (1983) described a basic four-stage model, consisting of four sequential stages: engagement, differentiation, interpersonal work and termination. Although this research has taken place in verbal psychotherapy groups, findings can be applied to other types of groups.

The approach to DMP

There are points of reference that, if taken into consideration, help to involve participants in the active, creative rhythmic process of DMP more easily than if they were ignored.

The participants will need help to be in touch with their feelings as well as thoughts and to maintain a balance between the two. A carefully chosen structure and a directive approach need to be matched with open-ended spontaneity bringing in unintended practices as appropriate to facilitate the group's authentic expression.

In DMP your primary function is to help individuals find an acceptable identity and a more satisfying mode of behaviour for themselves. It is important to maintain a context of flow and focus between both inner and outer processes.

You will need to be sincere, offering genuine unconditional acceptance of the group's themes and behaviours, and to be empathic with their difficulties. There needs to be an expectancy of success and clear boundaries, including the setting of ground rules at the beginning of a group's life. The 'belief cycle'—where, if the group believes in you and you believe in your methods and medium, the two reinforce one another—creates a positive energy in the group and session as a whole. Eventually you can become more of a follower as the group itself takes the lead.

The activities or techniques utilised are only part of the session and should not be viewed as a panacea. No single method is ever effective for all groups, all difficulties or all practitioners/therapists. It is more important to give attention to the way the activities are used to encourage groups to believe in their own power to help themselves, to acknowledge and solve their own difficulties, to facilitate learning and to mobilise expectancy for success.

It is wise to put theory, method and technique to the back of your mind once you begin the session. It is the process that is in the 'here and now' that needs to be worked with; visualise your feet in contact with the earth to help your own grounding and improve spontaneity and authentic responses, whether they are verbal or non-verbal.

In DMP success will not be in the achievement of a particular movement task or phrase, although spin-offs do lie in the completion of, for example, a stretch jump or a controlled turn into a fall. These are important in the development of confidence in body capabilities and co-ordination, but for growth there needs to be a shift in emphasis from goal-oriented body/movement success to using movement and dance as a diagnostic tool and integrating force in the emotional–physical–social (biopsychosocial) arena.

You, as a psychotherapist, in using the activities as a vehicle to reach your goals/objectives, need to meet the group members at their level, then they may be able to initiate development to another level (however small the step) so they may grow in a personal way and any change reverberates through the whole self. By identifying ordinary movement behaviour and crystallizing the qualities in their movement, a recognition of the 'here and now' is brought about, together with the confidence to explore alternative movement as the process evolves towards transpersonal development. There is a balance between the 'here and now' and the 'then and there'.

In dance and movement there is a quality of impermanence linked to early stages of play, where the importance lies in doing, not producing. In dance, the movement is there, and then gone. This may feel safer for some people than methods that formalise and preserve the medium of expression facilitating their engagement.

Some suggestions for programme structure

1 Always practice within your limitations of training and experience.
2 Having collected your group together you may like to use movement observation (see pp. 82–89) and/or other observations of behaviour to develop some general aims and identify relevant activities. Base the first session on a variety of activities with the specific objective of assessment. Identify participants' strengths and needs in terms of movement, other non-verbal communication, verbalisation, self-disclosures, participation in the group and so on.
3 When planning the second session you need to build on group strengths rather than limitations, as working with preferred ways to begin with builds self-esteem and can support what may be very weak egos.
4 Ensure that the sessions are at a consistent time and place. You will need to decide whether to 'close' the group to other participants after the first or second session or to leave it as an 'open' group. You will need to be clear with everyone on the number of sessions you will meet for.
5 Use the programme gradually to plan ways in which less preferred ways of moving can be experienced to widen movement resources in the group. Develop variations in the activities to allow for this incorporation, then restructure, redefine and clarify goals for the sessions.
6 Share with others in the setting how the media of movement and dance can help, hinder and provoke

changes for the group. Be open to questions, while maintaining confidentiality.

7   Evaluate themes and movement as well as the emotional responses for both individuals and the group as a whole after each session. Reflect on your own style, interventions, feelings and speculations about the session.

8   Develop the resource of movement and dance for use within the treatment programme, specifically in socio-emotional aspects relevant to the organisation.

Anticipated outcomes

As a result of the intervention programme it is hoped participants will become more aware and will have internalised several skills and processes in order to fulfil their potential for growth. The following are two possible areas of awareness, with relevant dimensions.

Self-awareness

Sense of internal structure; reduction of impulsivity and perseveration; visualisation skills; imitation skills; self-disclosure; acknowledging and giving others feedback; development of body image, body awareness; wider movement range; isolation and articulation of body parts; adaptability; sensitivity to self; co-ordination skills; assertion skills; decision making. Emotional self-regulation, resilience and emotional intelligence are more recent aspects for attention that can be improved, especially from engagement with DMP.

Social awareness

Co-operation; conforming to a structure; waiting turn; empathy; giving feedback; sharing; leading, following; giving and receiving attention; appropriate physical contact; initiation of activity; group participation; leaving a group and you, the group leader.

Figure 2.3 **Evaluation sheet for a DMP session**

Amended from Payne (1981)

Date:

Session no:

Present:

Absent:

---

1   Time and length of session

2   Setting

3   Population

4   Props/music used and reasons

5   Themes predominant (movement and psychodynamic)
    a) Themes you arrived with

    b) Themes evolving from group

6   What happened overall (including structures used, responses and group dynamics)?

7   Any changes noted?

8   Any specific expressions?
    a) Verbal

    b) Non-verbal

9   Assessment (include socialisation skills related to objectives; objectives achieved; future objectives for next session).

10 Any other comments?

11 Your own process recording (what happened for you? Include any ideas, images, memories, feelings which emerged for you before, during and after this group session).

Forms of evaluation

Your evaluation of the group may take place both after each session (formative) and at the end of the programme (summative). It will always need to refer back to the specific goals and general aims you articulated at the outset. Figure 2.3 is an example of a structure for formative evaluation and has been used in practice.

Four sample sessions

The following examples show how a session might be planned for, with overall aims that develop from perceived needs or educational or treatment goals. The session's objectives arise from the previous session, and the theme is introduced and developed in accordance with these objectives. It is important to remember that the activities can be amended to respond to different needs, overall aims and session objectives, and that there are no pre-scriptive formulae guaranteed to remedy specific difficulties or engender particular responses with any one population.

The following sample sessions are examples of work that has actually taken place; the preliminary session plans have been amended retrospectively to illustrate what actually took place and worked. All the activities have been tried and tested over time; however, they will be affected by the style and manner in which they are presented; only you will be able to adapt them to suit your groups and yourself. The term 'leader' replaces the terms either 'psychotherapist' or 'practitioner' for ease of reference.

The sessions are taken from work in the following settings:

1 special school (young children);
2 community home (older children);
3 young people's unit (adolescents);
4 summer school workshop (adults).

The groups include both verbal and non-verbal clients, with labels such as 'moderate and severe learning difficulties', 'autistic', 'child depressive', 'young offender', 'school phobic' and 'normal neurotic'.

Example 1 Special school *Department of non-communi cating children (young children assessed as autistic/ psychotic)*

Overall aims:

▶ To assess then select four groups, out of 16 children, diagnosing needs, taking into account their overall treatment/educational programme aims.

Session objectives:

▶ To assess the needs of each group member in terms of physical development/capability and relationship.
▶ To assess the helper's role and potential working rela- tionship with each group member; particular attention will be paid to the helper's ease/unease with the movement activities.
▶ To assess members' use of space, awareness of body parts, rhythm, body actions and touch.

Session number 1:

▶ (From a 1-year programme, reviewed intermittently.)

Number in group:

▶ Nine, including four helpers—all previously known to each other, having worked together in other treatment programmes. The group practitioner/therapist is also well known to all members. This is the first of three groups that are taking part in the initial assessment sessions.

Duration of session:

▶ 45 mins

Gender:

▶ Mixed

Equipment:

▶ Mats
▶ Sticky-backed white tape on floor, making lines.

Warm-up

1 Removing shoes and socks at the edge of the room with help from the helpers, leader (practitioner/therapist) says hello to each child and spends some time verbally preparing them for the movement session.
2 Sitting on the white line at the edge of the space, shuffling selves on seats, pushing with hands, over the line, forward and backward as a group. Repeat with rhythmical singing accompaniment: 'We can push ourselves forward, we can push ourselves backward.'

Introduction to theme

1 Each in turn is given a ride by the helper, who stands up to pull the children along the floor on their backs. They move away from the line so that they can still see the group, and then back again. Show helpers how to hold wrists for a firm grip and to use their legs, not backs, to pull. Perhaps sing the child's name and a song saying they are having a ride for each.

2 All at the same time given a pulling ride along floor (corner to corner).
3 In a circle, sitting, hands touching hands, feet, knees, clapping, feet stamping, all to a singing accompaniment.

Development of theme

1 All moving out of circle and into circle on seats, moving in, arriving and clapping, moving out and stamping.
2 Rocking onto backs with feet going high above heads, coming back to centre and clap, clap, clap; again, singing accompaniment.
3 Individually, in own space, helper rolls child in a long-stretched shape, all crawl back to centre of space.
4 In twos, hand to hand, long rolling together to a corner and running back to centre.

Warm-down

1 Sitting in a partner's lap, enjoy a slow rock, reverse roles.
2 Creeping slowly back to the edge of the space find your shoes and socks and put them on.
3 Leader goes and sits and says goodbye to each person in turn.

What follows is an extract from the author's notes for this session which may help to illustrate how the session went, what was evaluated and adjustments decided upon for the succeeding sessions.

When I asked for shoes and socks to be removed this caused some upset for both helpers and children. They were unprepared for this, they expected to work in their shoes, the helpers especially. I need to brief helpers prior to sessions of my expectations and any difficulties they can envisage. I felt very unsure of my ground immediately, I felt this requirement was me forcing my standards upon non-movement orientated people. For the children this was establishing a new routine and one which demanded quite some time to complete. I felt useless only saying hello, so I also helped each helper to remove children's shoes and socks. This made me feel less nervous and framed my 'hellos'.

We sat on the line, all except B who would not, despite lots of encouragement from me and her helper. I felt she was being stubborn; I left her to stand and concentrated on the others, sitting down with them. She seemed very powerful, her tall body overseeing us all. After a minute she joined us sitting. None of them could comprehend directions and all found the floor work difficult, often wanting to stand and run off. It was hard work just to acknowledge their fear and need to escape the containment by separating from the ground and the group. The pushing–slithering was not successful at this stage. The pulling rides were, perhaps because they could feel the physical sensation of the floor in contact with their body more easily as it moved across the floor by an external force, rather than self-initiated. They were able to tolerate touch at this level. The rides from corner to corner were inappropriate—too much space for them to feel secure, too frightening. Perhaps they need to be in a more limited space to concentrate on body awareness through surfaces and rolling action. In future, all floor work needs to involve body awareness and task centred activities (such as moving on hands and knees, elbows and knees, knees only). Contrary to my belief, it seems best not to change the activity too quickly but stick to one for a longer time, modifying it very slightly as it progresses. This was a surprise to me. I thought they would need to change very quickly from one activity to another because of attention spans and interest levels being so limited. Their motor skills, developmentally, were not good but adequate to continue with the floor as their basic support, with a helper. Running was by far the favourite activity—this they nearly all managed very well! Rocking feet over heads was very successful, perhaps the sensation of the rock is exciting, some members are very competent at this on their chairs or on their feet as a ritualized personal movement. Moving in and out of the circle seemed too difficult—not enough boundaries, again lost in space perhaps. More time needed for initial group interactions from the line to the circle formation, possibly leave circle work to the end in future.

Rolling the child was enjoyed by all, but upon my suggestion for the child to roll the helper, although the children were delighted the helpers seemed to feel very vulnerable. They were not used to receiving in this way from the children very often, they may have felt out of control. I will need to bear this in mind when planning the programme. T would not be rolled but did roll his helper, perhaps it appealed to his need to be powerful. Helper J said he would like to be rolled but could not allow it. Something here about letting go of control, being passive to allow self to be rolled. I was also being rolled by a member, which had the disadvantage of my not being in control of the group, not able to hold the space for them; but the advantage of letting helpers and children see me as a model and as able to let go in this way. (Generally, I acted as partner to one of the children.) M very excited, particularly in hand to hand rolling especially when near to the edge of the space, F competent at rolling, rocking and clapping. S seemed afraid to roll onto her front—lots of grimaces of pain. She could only clap once, a soft one, seemed timid throughout session. It felt like she was made of glass, very fragile. There was no synchronous movement or claps/stamps.

Assessment conclusions in relation to some session objectives

1 Brief helpers on movement tasks planned for session.
2 Plan programme around:
   a body parts (hands meeting and parting; knees to chin, etc.);
   b rhythm (singing, claps and stamps to accompany movement with helpers—not in large group);
   c space (task centred to mat/line);

    d   body actions (pushing along on seats, rolling);
    e   touch (in contact work such as rocking/rolling).

3   Split group into two comprised of: S, M, F/T, B (able and less able mixed together).

4   Child–helper in a one-to-one relationship (J + S, P + M, R + F, J/L + T).

Example 2 Community home (*older children, in care*)

Overall aims:

▶ The same as the home had identified for each child referred, for example (a) to come to terms with leaving the institution; (b) to reduce anxiety and aggression levels.

Session objectives:

▶ To reduce impulsivity.
▶ To work in pairs.
▶ To acknowledge their need to compete with each other.

Duration of session:

▶ 1 hour

Session number:

▶ 16 (out of a series of 42)

Number in group:

▶ Six

Gender:

▶ Male

Equipment:

▶ Mat per child
▶ Music (MP3 playlists/CDs)
▶ Drums and other percussion

Warm-up

The leader (practitioner or therapist) counts from one to five and group have to run to touch two walls and return to the centre mat. Who can return first? The leader asks can they now beat their own record. Repeat. The leader asks who they would most like to beat. Repeat activity.

Introduction to theme

1   Leader allocates partners. In turn they follow and move as their partner does, while remaining on their mats (pushed together). Music of one duo's choice is used and the leader turns it off at random, when all have to freeze in stillness for two to three seconds. Movement sections need to be kept short to retain interest. The challenge is for the partner initiating the movement of their choice to make it difficult for their partner to follow. Leader tells the group to change initiators at varied intervals.
2   Leader asks each pair to select a piece of percussion. They use the percussion to accompany their partner's movement for about 30 seconds, when the leader says 'change' and roles are reversed. Partner moving can introduce stillness at any time; the percussionist has to wait until the mover moves again before playing. Challenge is for the mover to try to trick the player into playing while there is stillness. Mats in use to define space.
3   Using all the space the leader drums a beat for all to move to and then freeze when beat stops. Identify the movement activity from members' suggestions, eg.

running, leaping etc. At the leader's suggestion each member of the group uses drum for the activity.

4 Leader drums a beat for the group to gather energy and swing into a jump and freeze in a shape, gripping the floor firmly. Two members of group try to move each of the others from their spot, to leader's count of four.

Development of theme

1 In pairs of own choosing, mime any sport. Give 2 minutes for them to perfect this. Have them slow the mime down considerably but keeping the same overall pattern. Share each mime, with the others trying to guess the sport portrayed.

2 Leader uses the mime movement as a basis to lead the group in a dance. The group are asked to follow the leader's movement as closely as possible with their own. Each member is on their own mat, while being part of the circle. The leader contrasts the movement with opposite qualities/shapes. Music of their choice is used as an accompaniment (each member gets his choice at some point in the session). If feasible, after bringing the group dance to an end encourage each child in turn to use one of the mime movements to lead the group dance to begin again. After a short time suggest they bring it to an end in stillness.

3 In group discussion encourage each member to remember who they partnered and to say one thing they appreciated about their partner. Have each complete the sentence 'I did not expect ... ' and share it, ask them all how they would describe their behaviour during exercise/whole session.

Warm-down

Lying back on the floor, close eyes and breathe out four times. Tension-release exercise—leader names each body part in turn, beginning with feet and finishing with the face. Open eyes and slowly stand up.

Example 3 Young people's unit in a psychiatric hospital (*adolescents*)

Overall aims:

▶ Same as for their stay in the unit. For example (a) to see if they can become more confident in their body; (b) to offer a complementary experience to psycho-drama and verbal psychotherapy.

Session objectives:

▶ To reinforce levels of creativity.
▶ To be more aware of self in movement and the group.
▶ To explore the theme of power in both open and closed body shape.

Orientation:

▶ Non-sexist

Gender:

▶ Mixed

Duration:

▶ 50 minutes

Number in group:

▶ Eight (two staff helpers)

Session number:

▶ Six (in a series of 12)

Equipment:

▶ Music (MP3 playlists/CDs)
▶ Drum

Warm-up

1 In circle, exercises using stretches forward and side; straightening and bending knees; twisting spine and rising and sinking of whole body. Each repeated four times to music of their choice.
2 In twos, name game using hand gesture to say how they feel today, then repeating saying their name with the same gesture.
3 In circle, whole group repeats name and gesture three times, after each in turn.
4 Leader develops a group movement using the gestures as a basis, exaggerating them and linking them together in a rhythmical pattern. The group move with the leader, following the patterns.

Introduction to theme

In own space; individually close all of the spaces between your body parts and between you and the floor. Make your body feel very closed and tight. Helpers try to 'undo' them, without success. Now make as much space as you can between body parts (can vary the speed with which this is done). Notice the difference; any words to describe this shaping? Standing up, walk across space in your usual manner. Now repeat with tight body shapes and open shapes alternately; which feels familiar to some extent? Discuss in pairs how it felt to do this and to what extent you were aware of your normal shaping.

Development of theme

1   In pairs, A sculpts their partner, B, into the shape they are aware B normally adopts; is it mainly open or wide, or taking up little space? If you do not know, ask B if they are aware. Now exaggerate the shape so that it is more open or closed. Then sculpt them into the opposite shape; ask them for one word that describes how that feels. Go around to look at the other people's shapes, for 30 seconds. Return to partner and tell each other what you experienced, for 2 minutes. Change roles.

2   With a different partner, sitting back to back, knees up, hands on floor—a competition to push partner across space. Leader beats drum for a short time, they freeze when drumbeat ceases. Now a new partner: one pushes, the other receives the push and guides the direction of travel. Drumbeat. Reverse roles. Discuss how it was to be the pushed and the pusher. Which is the more familiar to you? Give group members a turn on the drum.

3   In the large group, leader asks members: 'Select for yourself one person whom you sense is the opposite from the way you feel you are at the moment. In turn say to them why you think that (no response need be made from them). Try to relate it to how you see them sit/stand/move in the unit. It does not matter if you do not find an opposite, you may like to comment on how you see yourself in terms of body shape.' The leader may need to encourage this feedback and to keep the time strictly, e.g. spending no more than 3 minutes.

Warm-down

1   Leader asks for comments on which exercise felt difficult and which felt safe to do. Perhaps ask for them to reflect on what habits have come to their attention today in themselves and others.

2   Return to the shape your partner sculpted you into earlier, move around the room with an awareness of how this feels, taking it up, then moving on alternately.

3 Close eyes and breathe out, noticing the noises outside the room, then those here, especially their own breathing. Slowly, in time with their own breath, open eyes.

Example 4 Summer school *as part of summer school workshops* (*adults*)

Overall aim:

▶ To introduce the use of creative dance for self-awareness and as a process for the self-development of their client groups.

Session objectives:

▶ To create a sense of trust in the group.
▶ To aim to overcome some members' inhibitions about movement.
▶ To develop group cohesion.

Duration of session:

▶ 2 hours

Number in group:

▶ 16

Gender:

▶ Mixed

Session number:

▶ Two (in a series of five)

Equipment:

▶ Music (MP3 playlists/CDs)
▶ Parachute

Warm-up

In a circle, each member leads the warm-up, starting with the leader, taking turns spontaneously. They are asked to name a body part they sense as needing to move and to lead the group in a simple movement for that part. Repeat movement eight times to some gentle/lively music of their choosing.

Introduction to theme

1   In pairs, one in front of the other, the first with their eyes closed and forearms up as if the headlights of a car. The one behind will guide them by the arms slowly around the space, changing speed, direction, stopping and reversing. Move them as if they are an old car, going uphill, round roundabouts, at traffic lights, turning right and left. Then the leader suggests that they are as if on a motorway, can go faster yet still take good care of their car and avoid others. The leader can direct the tasks as their confidence grows, for 5 to 10 minutes, with a change of roles at intervals.

2   Give a new partner a spin, a ride on your back (need to teach safe support), a lean on you. Change roles. With a new partner again, stand up and sit down together, so sharing your weight with each other sensitively.

3   In threes, trust exercises as in activity 'Relationship 13', p. 267.

4   Groups of four or five, as in activity 'Relationship 11', p. 265.

5   Groups of six or seven, as in activity 'Relationship 6', p. 260.

Development of theme

1 As in activity 'Relationship 12', p. 266.
2 Leader presents parachute to the group as a whole, requesting that they unfold it and work with it as a group for 10 minutes. Ask if they would like music; if so, ensure that it is long enough and not overly demanding in energy all of the time. Suggest that they each take it in turn to initiate a movement, beginning with yourself, then name each person, going round the circle. After a while suggest each take a space for themselves to do a special 'trick'. Finally suggest they have one more turn, spontaneously, leading the group, the leader asking for one to lead a closing movement. Perhaps then ask for comments on their experience of the group dance.

Warm-down

As in 'Relationship 13', p. 267.

Clients

Some groups require special attention and need placement in rehabilitative, educative or health settings. The reasons are varied. In this text we are concerned with those populations who display behaviour that does not adequately satisfy their needs, and/or is demonstrating a lack of adjustment to the demands of their environment. The labels given to such groups may vary. They include 'at risk', 'emotionally and behaviourally disturbed', 'disaffected', 'socially disadvantaged', 'delinquent', 'personality or conduct disordered' and 'problematic', and many are labelled 'psychiatrically disturbed', 'learning disabled' and so on. They may also present with a physical, sensory, linguistic or cognitive handicap.

Having said that, all of us can grow and become more aware if we choose. Humanistic psychology reminds us of this. People do not have to be labelled or in institutions to be in need of opportunities for personal development. This is the reason for including a 'normal' adult group in the sample sessions above. The group was attending a workshop as part of a summer school that focused on all the arts therapies: the group was self-selected, and most group members were either professionals in one of the helping services or interested artists.

We can, however, make some general assumptions about our clients.

1   A group member's reaction to a space, leader and other participants will, to some extent, be a manifestation of their response in other situations.
2   Every participant is special and can change to extend their potential within the context of the session. Flexibility of response to the emotional and physical demands of life is possible.
3   Opportunities are needed for the individual to learn about themselves in a safe, structured and yet exploratory setting.
4   Dance and movement experiences are one way of re-educating the patterned emotional–physical responses. The purpose is to recover the ability to choose how to live in a positive manner acceptable both to the individual and to society (the implication being that the individual needs to be able to handle society creatively, rather than being pressured into conforming).
5   Movement and dance activities as experiences for growth provide a vehicle for:

    a   the establishment of individual identity;
    b   social learning in the opportunities for exploration of generalisable alternative behaviours.

Laban movement analysis

In this material we are concerned with creative dance and movement as means of supporting groups with specific needs, often vulnerable, to become, for example, more skillful, raise their self-esteem, increase well-being and quality of life. The use of creative dance and movement as a psychotherapy aims to help groups with a disturbance and/or disability to organise and develop a repertoire of behaviour that will enable them to satisfy their own needs and adjust more adequately to the demands of their environment. This transformation arises from working at a body–movement as well as emotional and learning levels. Since we are working with both the body and the mind system of language, which can help identify and clarify movement themes, objectives and observations are important.

Laban's contributions were both in the promoting of creative dance and in his system for observing and categorising movement. In this system attention is shifted towards the vocabulary, analysis and observation of movement: what we move (body), how we move (effort), where we move (space) and with what or whom we move (relationship).

By observing through these categories, we become sensitised to the range of movement behaviour people have, their strengths and limitations expressed as 'effort habits' and 'shaping preferences'. From this information (and an assessment of behavioural aspects as gained through tests, observation charts and checklists) a programme of dance and movement sessions relevant to the person's needs can be developed.

Laban viewed movement holistically, as a process—the fragments of body, effort, space and relationships added together do not make the whole; the whole is greater than the parts that are combined together. Movement is only a part of behaviour, but in observing and describing or defining it we can be aware of the variation within that behaviour. The reintegrative process can be helped without verbal acknowledgement by client or therapist, through gradual or sudden changes in the movement. However, it must not be a prescriptive or 'filling in the gaps' approach, such as might be found in rote learning or imposed dance exercises that are isolated from the total organism. These are 'conditioned' responses and are not spontaneous or authentic in the multi-level process.

There is no need for psychological training to decode messages communicated non-verbally (e.g. a depressed posture), nor is specific training needed to be aware of a person's physical presence, which could be strengthened by moving experiences in re-education. Sensitivity as a mover, group leader and observer are required, however, and courses may help to heighten this awareness (see Section 4, 'Training in dance movement psychotherapy'). There are cross-cultural variants that need to be contextualised, for example when working with multi-ethnic groups (Blacking, 1977).

Movement observation is valuable in three ways:

1   as a tool for identifying the individual movement strengths and limitations; movement observations are only a starting-point and should be pooled with other information before assessing the needs and developing a relevant programme;
2   as a device that enables you to observe the client outside the confines of other relationships;
3   as a method of identifying movement themes and the setting of movement goals for the group within the session.

Laban movement analysis (LMA) may be employed to encourage variability and range of movement with reference to what part of the body moves, the bodily action, movement quantities, and the use of shape or space. The summary below can support the development of an activity to focus on a different aspect of movement, be it action, level, quality, what is to be moved etc. The activities supplied in this book can be varied to promote a greater range of movement for clients cultivating flexibility as opposed to rigidity, balance as opposed to imbalance, leading to a spectrum of capacities and a widening and deepening of bodily experiences. In today's sedentary society it is important to engage people in activity to connect with their vitality. Creative, active and relational movement provides a basis for developing inter- and intra-personal skills, thinking, emotional intelligence, self-regulation and overall well-being.

A summary of LMA is given below.

What moves

This is the 'body' as a whole, its different parts in isolation and in co-ordination.

Shapes in movement or stillness

a   curled
b   stretched
c   wide
d   twisted

(see Glossary).

Activity
Locomotion, elevation, turns, gestures, stepping, stillness.

Body parts
Knees, arms, hands, head etc.

Symmetry
Both sides of the body doing the same thing simultaneously (see Glossary).

Asymmetry
One side of the body moving independently and/or differently from the other.

Body flow
Successive or simultaneous; peripheral or central. Body parts initiating/leading movement.

How the body moves

This is the quality of the movement termed 'effort', comprised of a combination of factors (dynamics and textures) conveying our inner attitudes, thoughts and feelings. There are four main factors:

Time
Revealed through suddenness (sharp, quick, urgent) and sustainment (prolonged, unhurried, slow).

Weight
Revealed by the degree of muscular tension varying between firm (forceful, resistant, strong) and light (delicate, gentle, buoyant).

Space
Identifies the extent to which a movement is generous or economic in the use of space—it may be between extremes of directness (undeviating, straight) and flexibility (indirect, roundabout). This is not to be confused with *where the body moves.*

Flow
This factor concerns the freedom of flow or restraint with which a movement is carried out, the extremes being free, fluent, easy and ongoing movement that can only be stopped with difficulty, and tightly controlled, bound, restricted movement that can easily be stopped at any point in its journey.

NB. It is a combination of these 'efforts' that make vehicles for our feelings.

Where the body moves—space

Personal space
This is the space into which we move, immediately surrounding the body. *Inner space*: That which is contained inside our bodies.

General space
That which is outside the immediate reach, where we find ourselves, e.g. corridor/ward/hall/playground. We move into general space taking our personal space with us.
Levels
High, medium and low. Movement takes place at any of these levels and in different directions (see Glossary).
Directions
Forward, backward, to one side and the other, upwards and downwards and all the way around. *Diagonals* are a combination of these (see Glossary).
Extension into space
Near or far.
Air and floor pathways
Curved/straight patterns can be carved out of the air and on the floor with gestures or whole body (see Glossary).
Space actions
Rise—sink/open—close/advance—retreat.

With whom or what we move—relationship (see Glossary)

Relatedness of body parts to each other, relationship to self.

Relationship of individuals to each other.

Relationship of groups to each other.

Relationship to environment: objects, space.

Relationship implies the world of people, objects and stimuli with whom and with which we live, work and play. It implies listening, watching, initiating or responding to contact. *Body* (what), *effort* (how) and *space* (where) all hinge upon the core issue of *relationship*, without which growth would not take place.

By extracting the major areas of LMA, some possible starting-points can be illustrated diagrammatically (see Figure 2.4). The idea is that each area is connected yet grows out

Figure 2.4 **Laban Movement Analysis as a starting point for developing activities**

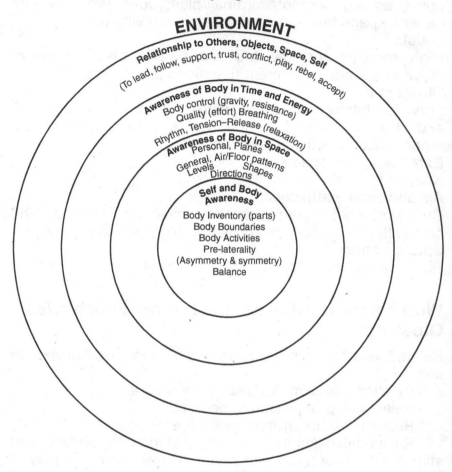

ENVIRONMENT
Relationship to Others, Objects, Space, Self
(To lead, follow, support, trust, conflict, play, rebel, accept)

Awareness of Body in Time and Energy
Body control (gravity, resistance)
Quality (effort) Breathing
Rhythm, Tension–Release (relaxation)

Awareness of Body in Space
Personal, Planes
General, Air/Floor patterns
Levels   Shapes
Directions

Self and Body Awareness
Body Inventory (parts)
Body Boundaries
Body Activities
Pre-laterality
(Asymmetry & symmetry)
Balance

of the whole. The emphasis of the experience offered may only be in one area, however. The figure gives an overall picture of the way each aspect can be viewed as inter-related, layer upon layer. Supplementary aspects have been included where they are thought to be particularly relevant to groupwork, for example 'Breathing', 'Rhythm', 'Body boundaries' (see Glossary) and 'Pre-laterality'.

Guidelines for you

Personal preparation for session

The following points may be useful to you, particularly when working with very difficult groups, whether in DMP or in another context using creative dance and movement with other intentions.

1 Rehearse and visualise where, with whom, and how the session will take place.
2 Look at your apprehensions/fears for the sessions, for example your feelings about your own body and movement and acceptance of the work with colleagues. How will you overcome these?
3 What do you expect to go well in the session?
4 What will be the most difficult problem? What strategy will you use to overcome it?
5 Decide on the minimum response from the group that you will be satisfied with.
6 What do you think the group needs as a minimum response to feel satisfied?
7 Read through your evaluation notes from the previous session and plan for this one.
8 Put the plan to the back of your mind so that you can be open to responses from within the group. Be prepared to shape your plan around relevant themes emerging.
9 Think about what equipment you require, and its collection. Can it be used safely in the space? When will you use it?
10 How will you finish?
11 Immediately prior to the session, centre yourself in a quiet place, alone.

Hints on the environment

A structured, safe environment gives an opportunity to participate in the movement dialogue with the leader or others, using latent and manifest sources of movement symbolism to understand and recognise how they conduct their life and how they can alter it.

It may be best to start with a small space: a classroom, music room, meeting place etc. You need to be sure that this can be used exclusively by your group during the session time; interruptions can be very disturbing to any groupwork. You may need to be prepared for clients to have some associations with the space prior to your session, for example as a place for talking, playing, being quiet, doing schoolwork, or being in another type of group or activity.

Some noise may be made in your group, so you may need to find out if this would cause anyone else outside the session inconvenience and, if so, to negotiate for a relocation and so on.

A large gymnasium or hall may prove threatening and overwhelming to your group. If this is the only space available, try sectioning it off with benches, tables and mats.

Be aware of any distractions in the space (e.g. hanging mobiles, mirrors, pictures, books, instruments, mobile phones). Remove these whenever possible and ensure that the space remains consistent over time, both in its internal decoration and in its availability, to promote added security for the groups.

You need to keep the space sparsely furnished and the floor clean. Carpets tend to be an inhibition to movement and nylon carpets are positively dangerous. Small mats, cushions or chairs could be used for the beginning or end of the session, if felt appropriate, to focus the group. For some populations, for example those with a physical handicap, the elderly or those in long-stay psychiatric care, chairs may need to be kept as their base throughout the session, especially at first. Certainly for reflective discussion times cushions are often more comfortable for some groups. Mats are ideal for discussions and other activities you may wish to try. Small and light gym mats or yoga/exercise mats are best.

Encourage the group to remove shoes and socks at the start of each session, and insist on loose clothing. Have a laptop with your music playlist or a mobile phone and speaker to play music nearby and encourage participants to suggest music they like to move to.

Working with colleagues

When working with other staff in the group you need to ensure that you have negotiated expectations with each other. For the physically less able, sensitive and supportive help from other members of your team (e.g. a physiotherapist) may be useful. It is invaluable to have evaluation and planning communications between numerous different colleagues. In this way the programme may be designed from shared information in the interest of all group members and may be congruent with the establishment's overall aims/rehabilitation programme. You need to be prepared to translate your work into a vocabulary colleagues can understand.

Guidelines for sessional psychotherapists attempting an intervention programme of DMP

(Adapted from material first published in Payne, 1988.)

While the following points may seem obvious, they appear as guidelines; they can be disregarded or disagreed with, especially if you feel intuitively that they are not a good idea for your clients or yourself in your setting.

1   You will need to be clear about your aims and objectives and how you plan to implement them.

2   Spend time liaising with the senior leadership team of the establishment and other relevant health or education professionals (SENCo—special educational needs coordinator; educational/clinical psychologist) first, explaining the project and eliciting their advice/prejudices/biases, if any. Ask them to champion the group.

3   You may wish to give a presentation to all staff, outlining the project and focusing on the need for their full co-operation and support. Do not promise or guarantee anything; there is a tendency for staff to believe that the 'outsider' holds a magic formula and will change 'bad' behaviour into 'good' overnight. Explain any benefits that have taken place, however, as a result of research or previous programmes.

4   It may be desirable to give a demonstration session to the potential clients and staff. As a result of this, volunteers may come forward, willing to participate in the project. Limit numbers to between four and eight per group, although the numbers will be dependent on levels of functioning.

5   You will need to be careful about what you tell the clients and staff about the sessions—the words you use and the information you give will be determining factors in the attitude they will present about sessions. For example, with male adolescents labelled 'offenders' the sessions may be called 'movement' or just 'sessions' rather than 'dance', which could avoid stereotypes in their minds and those of the staff.

6   You need to be aware of the institutional philosophy, time management, organisational resistance and so on. You may need to adapt your programme to fit in with this in order to avoid conflict and confusion for staff and clients.

7   Consider how you might evaluate outcomes from a baseline before and after the group programme such as quality of life, well-being, symptom distress, anxiety, depression. There are measurement tools available for

all of these. You may be able to conduct a follow up to see if the outcomes are sustainable over time. Consider using an arts-based method, which might be more suitable for some clients than completing forms, even when these are part of an informal chat.

Support group for you

Many of the enquiries received by the ADMP (see Section 4) come from people interested in beginning work in the field or already quietly involving themselves in using dance and movement in establishments with various populations all over the UK. There seems to be an overwhelming need for contact with others who are working in a similar way.

In addition, people seem to need reassurance that what they are doing with their groups or individuals is 'OK': that is, it can be understood and has some value in its own right. They also need contact and support, and an opportunity to share work difficulties and to consult with others—outside their work setting—about their groups and sessions.

The ADMP came into being to meet just such a need (Payne, 1983, 1985). A small group of individuals met regularly in London to discuss their work, to tease out theoretical issues as they arose, and above all to 'move' together. This 'support group', as it was now termed, met for several years and gradually grew into what is now known formally as the ADMP. This, however, was the spin-off; the underlying desire was that need for support.

A support group can be seen to have five main objectives:

1   to make and maintain contact with others involved in, and sympathetic to, the use of dance and movement in groupwork;

2 to gain support for each other in what may be a vague and unknown area—and to work creatively together to overcome some of the difficulties in the work;
3 to explore other ideas in order to be useful to patients/clients: the support group is often a safe place to try out these ideas;
4 to create dancing experiences for each other and relate these to groupwork/client populations;
5 to prevent burn-out and isolation in what can be an extremely demanding profession sometimes.

Guidelines for your support group meeting

If you wish to form or be part of a support group, the following are points that may be used, changed or rejected as you see fit. All groups are different, and these guidelines may offer a springboard for some of them.

1 Ensure that you have each other's names, email addresses and mobile numbers.
2 Take it in turns to be the 'contact person' to arrange suitable days/times for meetings and to book the space.
3 If possible, meet centrally and in the same place. Church halls, drama halls, dance studios, colleges or schools may be suitable.
4 How often do you wish to meet? (This will depend on commitment, cost, place, group dynamics and so on.)
5 Do you wish to liaise with ADMP to gain members? (See 'Useful addresses'.) How large or small do you want the group to be? (Five to six members is often appropriate.)
6 What is the function of your group? What do you expect, what can you contribute, what are your hidden desires? How are you going to review the purpose of the group and its work?

7 Do you want to take it in turns to lead the group, experimenting with different activities and receiving feedback?

8 What topics do you wish to consider? These might include how to activate and motivate groups, safe and ethical practice, transference, resistance, touch, verbalisation, sexuality, creativity, use of video, sound and props, leaving a group.

9 Allow space for members to bring difficulties, finding a way to work with them as in role-play, or dancing out an issue based on a theme. One or two members may wish to watch, to give feedback on their perceptions of the process.

10 Are you going to share information gained from participation in relevant courses or workshops, reading lists, or have a loan system for articles or books?

11 Do you wish to visit each other's working environments? This may promote greater understanding of the context in which support group members work.

12 Make notes for yourself after each meeting.

13 What restrictions are there in your work? Can the group help you find creative ways of overcoming these?

14 Do you want to bring in outside leaders?

Remember that groups have their own dynamics. Stay with the work of the group, rather than exploring the dynamics of the group—that is, unless they really shout at you!

Supervision

The question of supervision often does not arise on the initial paths into this field. You may have colleagues or others to consult over issues, despite limitations of experience. However, the importance of supervision from experienced practitioners from outside any support group or work setting is vital. For professionals practicing DMP Payne (2008) provides different models of supervision and provides an overview of the topic.

In the UK, there are increasing numbers of experienced arts in health practitioners or dance movement psychotherapists able to offer supervision. Most dance movement psychotherapists are trained in supervision these days. If there is not one in your area, there may be a skilled practitioner who might be encouraged to offer you supervision on a regular basis. For the dance movement psychotherapist, preferably select an arts therapist or a body psychotherapist. Some of the problems arising in groupwork and in psychotherapy are universal: for example, finishing a programme of work, over-involvement and so on. These may all be issues you could discuss in relation to your own population. If you are still finding it difficult to find a suitable supervisor try a local psychotherapist (check the BACP/UKCP websites)—gestalt or another school/approach—they may be helpful for supervision (see Section 4 for some useful addresses).

Personal therapy

Concerning your own personal psychotherapy, this is now mandatory on the training programmes in the UK, although it can be the last thing to be considered for attention! Some people are quick and ready to offer themselves as psychotherapists, without having undergone any personal psychotherapy or groupwork.

Long-term intensive group or individual psychotherapy is as important as professional training and supervision for anyone intending to work or already working in DMP. Ideally, a DMP group itself would fit the bill. However, since experienced group-trained DMP practitioners are still scarce in the UK, especially outside the London bubble, one of the arts therapies, or group analytic, gestalt, psychodrama and other group approaches would serve. One-to-one therapies, including Reichian, transactional analysis, transpersonal/psychosynthesis or individual psychoanalysis (Jungian/Freudian) may be alternatives. However, if you intend to work with groups it is advisable to have had a group experience. It is very important to be discerning when selecting a psychotherapy and a psychotherapist. Be clear about what you want and feel good about the psychotherapist you have selected. (See Section 4 for some useful addresses. Please note that their inclusion is not to be perceived as recommendation.)

Conclusion

This section has covered the main theoretical aspects, including developmental movement processes, non-verbal communication, the facilitation of expressive dance and suggestions on the planning and evaluation of programmes. Four sample sessions served to illustrate some of the issues referred to in the text. LMA was presented for reference and some guidelines were suggested that may aid those new to the field in gaining some support for their work.

Helping clients to grow towards more healthy functioning through the use of creative dance and movement requires an approach that makes use of action and reflection. Through the use of movement observation skills to assess the type of intervention required, and the adaptation of a planned programme of work according to the changing needs of the group, participants will be able to engage with themes appropriate to their psychophysical stages of development. There needs to be a clear contract with the group and work setting that states whether the programme is psychotherapy or not. Those using the media of creative dance and movement need to be aware of the roles of practitioner and psychotherapist and to develop their own guidelines and support for setting up programmes of work.

SECTION 3

ACTIVITIES

INTRODUCTION

What follows is a sample of ideas for activities that have proven useful in practice with a variety of special needs groups, whether adults, young people or children. All have been developed in practice with a large range of populations in a spectrum of settings. For example, some have been employed with children with profound learning differences, others with high-functioning adolescents with an eating disorder and some with adults with a mental health condition. Thus, some of the activities will be too complex for lower-functioning populations and others too basic for higher-functioning groups. They will need to be adapted to be made suitable for your group, and to yourself to be within your limitations and professional training.

Some activities are suitable for groups beginning their journey together, others are for groups that are more established. You will know which are the most suitable for your group. For example, early on in a group's life perhaps select those focused on developing trust, group climate, cohesion and alliance. Furthermore, as the practitioner/therapist you will have the knowledge and understanding of your group's needs to select the most appropriate activities for them at any particular time. Consequently, each activity may be employed for either DMP or movement and dance as recreation, education or performance. The intention may be different and the way of weaving them into sessions will also be dissimilar, however they can be designed and shaped by you to respond flexibly to the group's needs whatever the contract or aims/objectives/anticipated outcomes.

It is important to view these activities as a starting-point and to integrate them as part of the overall programme that the clients are involved with, whatever the focus and context. The activities presented here will therefore need to be amended to relate to clients: specifically, to their intellectual, spiritual, physical and emotional developmental levels. They should not be used 'cold', as isolated exercises, as a 'fill-in', but as part of a pre-planned and integrated approach. They should also be amended depending on context, environment and the objectives for the group. For some groups some activities may need a system of scaffolding prior to implementing them.

It is wise to begin with the activity you feel most comfortable with; normally you will need to have experienced it yourself and to have practised or rehearsed it, in your support group perhaps.

The activities are divided into four sections:

Warm-up: which may be useful in the initial stages of a session.
Introduction to theme: which sets the scene for a particular movement idea or could reflect a group theme.
Development of theme: which is a more in-depth activity to take the group further into a particular idea.
Warm-down: which is for use in closing sessions and includes a physical warm down, time for group reflection and a grounding activity before the group leave.

Guidelines for physical safety

1   You will need to have some basic knowledge of how the body functions anatomically and physiologically before attempting to use movement with client groups (see Section 4 for institutions offering relevant courses).

2   Before embarking on a programme you will need to be aware of any group member who (a) presents a medical problem or (b) is on medication; either may affect their level of participation. This may require access to client files and discussion with the person responsible for the client; it may also require the negotiation of confidentiality before any such material is made available to you as group leader.

3 For all groups you will need to be aware of participants' physical limitations (e.g. heart problems).

4 Be particularly sensitive to the issue of physical contact as this will arise in most groups whether as part of the planned activities or spontaneously. The ADMP website has guidance for ethical practice, which includes touch (www.admp.org.uk). All dance movement psychotherapists must adhere to ADMP's code of professional practice, which can be downloaded from the website.

CRAB FOOTBALL

Aims: To warm up group physically, release energy
Population: Children/adolescents
Conditions: Early sessions; no violence
Time: 10 minutes
Equipment: Soft medium-size ball, goals (wide goal for less skilled group); playing area appropriate for fitness level of group
Structure: Two equal groups

■ **Activity**

1 Two teams identified and shooting ends given.
2 Everyone on all fours, stomachs uppermost; only pass or shoot with feet.
3 Play for 4–5 minutes each way.

■ **Supplementary development of activity**

1 Must make four passes before shooting.
2 Change size of playing area.

■ **Additional outcomes**

Competition.
Accepting boundaries.
Working as a group.

BODY SENSATION 1

Aim: To experience body sensations through movement
Population: All
Conditions: Safety element, regular stops to re-orientate
Time: 5 minutes
Equipment: None
Structure: Individual, pairs

■ Activity

1 Spin on the spot, feeling the air rushing past.
2 Spin with a partner; use a firm handgrip (e.g. wrist to wrist).
3 Notice how your body feels afterwards.

■ Supplementary development of activity

1 Swing arm through air.
2 Swing leg.
3 Walk, to jog, to sprint.

■ Additional outcomes

People become aware of the sensations in their body as they move quickly through the space. They become more in touch with their bodies through these exercises.

BODY SENSATION 2

Aims: To become more aware of the tensions in our bodies; to begin to release tension
Population: All
Conditions: None
Time: 5 minutes
Equipment: Drum
Structure: Individual

■ Activity

1 While lying on the floor in open position, let eyes close.
2 Leader talks through a count of 1 to 5, during which each member tenses their whole body, including face, and holds breath.
3 Count down from 5 to 1 and release tension built up.
4 Count down from 5 to 1 again for further release, using breath.
5 Repeat the above for specific body parts identified by group member.

■ Supplementary development of activity

1 Use drum for build-up of tension; build up slowly in a crescendo.
2 Tension could be expressed in contraction, extension or twisting of body.

■ Additional outcomes

Sense of the tension required and of excessive habitual tension that needs release. Quiet time can enable deep awareness of body.

See p. 296 for this activity used in another stage.

BALANCE 1

Aims: To develop self-control and body awareness
Population: All
Conditions: None
Time: 4–5 minutes
Equipment: Music if desired
Structure: Individually and large group

■ Activity

1   On spot in circle, move one isolated body part (for example, circling an arm). Leader begins by modelling movement.
2   After a few of these, give opportunity for participants to identify and articulate one body part in turn around the group. Say out loud the name of the body part and the type of articulation.

■ Supplementary development of activity

1   Move two body parts.
2   Move one body part while the rest of the body is in a specified shape, e.g. kneeling, sitting, legs astride.

■ Additional outcomes

1   Awareness in large group; turn-taking and following in rhythmic pattern.
2   Identification and articulation of body parts.

See p.146 for this activity used in another stage.

BALANCE 2

Aims: To develop control of body; to break 'rules'
Population: Children, adolescents, 'acting-out' adults
Conditions: Early sessions
Time: 5 minutes
Equipment: Drum
Structure: Individual

■ Activity

1 Group at one side of room.
2 Walk across room and stop very still when hear drum, which beats rhythmically. Aim is to continue walking when feel like it, while drum still playing. Since the overt 'rule' is to 'stay still until the drum stops', they must aim to break that rule. Leader to ensure they understand that the rule can be broken.
3 Hold stillness while drum continues.
4 Ask for volunteer to drum. They can make a guess at who will break the rule each time.

■ Supplementary development of activity

1 Repeat, but run across room.
2 Repeat, but slide on belly across room.
3 Leader turns back on the group while drumming, so cannot see group.

■ Additional outcomes

Acknowledgement that 'rule-breaking' is possible in this structure.

See p.149 for this activity used in another stage.

LOCOMOTION 1

Aims: To move in accordance with a set rhythm, travelling (see Glossary) in a co-ordinated, rhythmic experience
Population: Children, adults
Conditions: None
Time: 10 minutes
Equipment: Drum, music of your choice
Structure: Whole group as individuals, in partners, trios

■ Activity

1 Leader beats out a rhythm on the drum or puts on the music.
2 Leader varies the rhythm and calls out ways of travelling (e.g. walk, gallop, slide, jump, slither).

■ Supplementary development of activity

1 Join up with a partner and follow the pattern of travelling the partner selects, while leader continues to beat out a rhythm; then repeat, reversing roles.
2 Repeat in trios, small groups, periodically changing the person deciding the pattern.
3 Let a volunteer beat out rhythm on drum or select the music for the group.

■ Additional outcomes

1 More trust develops as the leader is accepted.
2 All members can initiate their own ideas for travelling within the safety of a clear rhythmic pattern.
3 The group learns to follow the lead from others and turn-taking is experienced in taking the lead.

See p. 203 for this activity used in another stage.

LOCOMOTION 2

Aim: To promote movement range in locomotion (see Glossary)

Population: All
Conditions: None
Time: 5–10 minutes
Equipment: Plentiful space
Structure: Whole group

■ **Activity**

1 Leader suggests group walk at normal pace around room, individuals changing directions at will.
2 Speed up walk to become a jog.
3 Speed up jog to become a run.
4 Slow down run to regain the jog.
5 Slow down jog to return to walk.
6 Slow down walk to become twice as slow.
7 Twice as slow again.
8 Twice as slow. Ensure in this final stage that the movement is very sustained, i.e. feet moving through the stages of walking and participants concentrating on the minute movement from one stage to the next as transfer of weight etc. takes place.

■ **Supplementary development of activity**

Repeat above, beginning with slow walk and increasing run, then sprinting.

LOCOMOTION 3

Aims: To accept outside structure, co-ordination, rhythmic experience
Population: Children, adults
Conditions: None
Time: 10 minutes
Equipment: Drum, music of your choice
Structure: Whole group as individuals, in pairs, threes

■ Activity

1 Leader beats out a rhythm on the drum or puts on the music.
2 The group move at a walk, gallop, slide, jump, slither (etc.) as instructed by the leader.

■ Supplementary development of activity

1 Can join up with a partner and follow in the pattern of locomotion partner selects, then reverse roles.
2 Repeat in threes, small groups.
3 A volunteer beats out the rhythm and/or selects the music.

■ Additional outcomes

1 More trust develops as the leader is accepted.
2 All members can initiate their ideas for locomotion within a clear rhythmic pattern.
3 Following and turn-taking are experienced.

BODY BOUNDARY 1

Aim: Awareness of physical boundaries
Population: Children
Conditions: First sessions
Time: 5 minutes
Equipment: None
Structure: Individual

■ Activity

On leader's signal all run to a specified part of the room and push against it (e.g. wall, centre of floor) using hands and arms for the count of five. Use all strength, wide base (i.e. legs apart, one leg in front of the other and knees bent if standing), grit teeth etc.

■ Supplementary development of activity

1 Push with backs or sides.
2 Push for a longer count.
3 Run and touch three or four places on the edge of the space and return to the centre within the count of five.

■ Additional outcomes

1 Knowledge of the physical space.
2 Energy is built up for session.

NAMEGAME 1

Aim: To learn names
Population: All
Conditions: None
Time: 10 minutes
Equipment: None
Structure: Group and pairs

■ Activity

1 Each says own name in turn around the circle.
2 Each says own name and adds an accompanying gesture.
3 Repeat step 2 above; after each person's contribution the group echo the name and gesture three times.

■ Supplementary development of activity

1 Go away and, individually, select two or three (leader stipulates) movements you liked doing from the previous group activity. Link them up. This is a sentence of movement—rehearse it.
2 Join with a partner and move your sentence. Partner has to guess the two or three names these movements were linked to.
3 Join up partner's movements and own to form a longer sentence.
4 Make the sentence of movement travel across the space.
5 Add sounds (e.g. the names) to the movement.
6 Share with another pair.

■ Additional outcomes

1 Linking movements together.
2 Performing a movement phrase for others.

NAMEGAME 2

Aim: To ground group in the present
Population: All
Conditions: Early in programme (first session)
Time: 10 minutes
Equipment: None
Structure: Whole group

■ **Activity**

1   In a group circle, say your name in turn around the circle.
2   Next say your name and one 'thing' you notice.
3   Next say your name and express in movement that noticed 'thing'.
4   Whole group then mirror back the movement made once.

■ **Supplementary development of activity**

Leader uses all their movements (and group echoes). Leader initiates and develops them to link together with accompanying music.

■ **Additional outcomes**

Recognise and learn the names of people in group.

NAMEGAME 3 (SILLY WALKS)

Aims: To promote travelling movement activity and creativity; to learn each other's names
Population: Adults
Conditions: First session
Time: 20 minutes
Equipment: None
Structure: Partners/whole group

■ Activity

1 Find a partner, exchange names and invent three different silly ways of walking. Share ideas with a partner.
2 With the same partner, stand opposite, say their name, and use one of the walks to change places. Repeat this, each using all three walks. (Start 5 or 6 feet apart, no physical contact.)
3 Find a new partner, exchange names. Repeat step 2, using the favourite walk so far.
4 Find another partner, exchange names. Repeat step 2, using the least favourite walk.
5 Find a final partner, exchange names. Repeat step 2, using the walk you have left out so far. Can you remember the names of the last three partners?

■ Supplementary development of activity

1 Make a large group circle, place yourself opposite your original partner. Check that you know their name.
2 Spontaneously, but in turns, say your partner's name and exchange places, using one of your walks.
3 Repeat this several times, so that all partners have exchanged places. The rest of the group is to notice the names as they are shouted out, as well as the way people walk.

4   When you think you know another person's name, shout that name out; they then have to change places with you. Each person is to use one of the invented silly walks from the original three.

■ Additional outcomes

The whole group will be able to recall and say at least three names from the group, and everybody's name if the development has been used; they will often remember people by their walks.

WARM-UP

SHAKING OUT

Aim: To identify physical sensations in body
Population: Children, adolescents, adults
Conditions: Any session
Time: 5–10 minutes
Equipment: None
Structure: Whole group, partners

■ Activity

1 Whole group in circle. Leader suggests they all shake out different body parts in turn. Can use similes, e.g. 'shaking off drops of water'. Always go from periphery towards centre of body, e.g. hand, lower arm to upper arm. Leader models.
2 After first part has been thoroughly shaken out, stop and ask participants to compare any sensations with those in parts not yet moved.
3 Allow people to mention any aspects that they notice in their own bodies, e.g. tingling or warmth in the energised arm, numbness in the non-activated arm.
4 Work through the whole body systematically. Could sing an accompaniment to the exercise if appropriate.

■ Supplementary development of activity

Partners shake out some body parts, e.g. feet, legs.

■ Additional outcomes

1 The participants become aware of own bodies and their physical sensations.
2 Focus is on the body—sets the scene for rest of session.

BODY CONTROL 1

Aims: To reduce impulsivity and perseveration
Population: Children
Conditions: None
Time: 3 minutes
Equipment: Drum
Structure: Individual

■ Activity

1 Suggest the group move very quickly all over the space to drumming.
2 When drum stops they freeze and hold position.
3 Repeat freezing in different position each time.

■ Supplementary development of activity

1 Use drum as signal to stop—i.e. when drum is banged, freeze.
2 Have volunteer play drum.

■ Additional outcomes

Offers opportunity to control body from movement to stillness.

BODY CONTROL 2

Aim: Introduce idea of assertion in body shape and energy
Population: All
Conditions: Warmed-up joints
Time: 2 minutes
Equipment: Drum
Structure: Individual

■ Activity

1 Using a drum as accompaniment, leader suggests participants run and jump and finish in a strong shape—tall, wide, twisted, angular, rounded.
2 Select someone to help you to attempt to push the members to see how strongly they can hold their shape.
3 Ensure that the group use wide bases and bend at the knees in their shapes to resist the attempts at pushing them over by the volunteer.
4 Repeat with the suggestion of a different shape each time.

■ Supplementary development of activity

1 Extend the above by adding:

   (a) a half-fall,
   (b) a turn or
   (c) a movement
  after the shaping in stillness.

2 Volunteer could accompany with a drum.

■ Additional outcomes

Phrasing and combining movement forms.

FLOOR PATTERN 1

Aim: To develop adaptability on moving across the floor
Population: All
Conditions: None
Time: 3–4 minutes
Equipment: Lively, rhythmical music
Structure: Individual, partner

■ **Activity**

1 Explore patterns and shapes across floor using feet to step them out (participants can choose their own patterns and shapes or leader can give examples).
2 Each make up a step pattern that carves out a shape on the floor.
3 Repeat, but using music to accompany patterning.
4 Repeat the pattern, making the movement smaller/larger, covering whole of the floor space.

■ **Supplementary development of activity**

1 Follow a partner's step pattern and repeat.
2 Teach pattern to partner and step out both patterns together.

FLOOR PATTERN 2

Aim: To experience leading and following as a linked group
Population: Adults, children (adolescents if stick or material used instead of hand-holding)
Conditions: None
Time: 3–4 minutes
Equipment: None
Structure: Whole group

■ Activity

1 The group make a line, holding hands. Designate one of the people on the end as leader.
2 For one minute they walk, twisting and coiling like a snake, following the leader around the space.
3 Reverse this sequence of movements as near as possible, following the person at the other end of line as the leader.
4 Repeat with a new leader and a different method of travel, for example zigzagging.
5 Ask for a volunteer, who then separates from the group.
6 The group continue but make their line into a knot, travelling around and under each other; when thoroughly knotted they freeze, but at no time unclasp hands.
7 The volunteer then attempts to untie the knot by physically maneouvring the group.

■ Supplementary development of activity

1 Volunteer undoes knot by giving verbal instructions only to group.
2 Group undo own knot non-verbally.

■ Additional outcomes

Physical contact is engendered.

See p. 295 for this activity used in another stage.

LEVEL 1

Aim: To promote range of movement between the three levels (see Glossary)
Population: Children
Conditions: None
Time: 5 minutes
Equipment: None
Structure: Individually, pairs

■ Activity

1 Turn or spin at low level (i.e. on floor), for example on stomach, curled up on back, or sitting.
2 Turn or spin at medium level, e.g. on knees.
3 Turn or spin at high level, e.g. in a jump, on toes.
4 Leader to specify body parts taking the weight at first, then encouraging participants to find own.

■ Supplementary development of activity

1 Find a partner and turn or spin together; assist each other to explore moving at each level, with different body parts taking the weight.
2 Make up a movement phrase together where each level is explored within turning or spinning movement.

■ Additional outcomes

1 Adaptability within specific body activities of turning/ spinning.
2 Awareness of the three levels of movement.

VOCAL

Aim: To encourage sound and movement in combination
Population: Adults
Conditions: None
Time: 5–10 minutes (supplementary activity 20–30 minutes)
Equipment: None
Structure: Whole group

■ Activity

1 Suggest participants inhale through their nose, take a deep breath and hum it out softly together.
2 Repeat with a louder hum until breath fully exhaled.
3 Repeat using sounds; 'ah, ooh, ee, la, ba, ra, ha, om'.
4 Use one of the sounds to initiate movement on the out breath.

■ Supplementary development of activity

1
(a) Move from the sound 'la' and the base of the spine.
(b) Move from the sound 'ba' and the centre of the body (below the navel).
(c) Move from the sound 'ra' and the solar plexus (just above the navel).
(d) Move from the sound 'ya' and the heart area of the body.
(e) Move from the sound 'ha' and the throat area.
(f) Move from the sound 'ah' and the middle of the brow area.
(g) Move from the sound 'om' and the crown (top of the head).

2 Reverse the exercise above from (g) to (a).
3 Notice any images or colours that are associated with the sound/movement.

■ Additional outcomes

Control of breath and sound.

BREATH 1

Aim: To focus on the out breath
Population: All
Conditions: None—used as a prerequisite for vocal work
Time: 2–3 minutes
Equipment: None
Structure: Whole group

■ **Activity**

1 Group stand in a circle—look towards the floor centre.
2 Leader suggests they close eyes and make a deep breath out.
3 Relax shoulders, arms and legs; bend slightly at the knees.
4 Allow breath to drift out slowly through the nose.
5 Repeat, allowing breath to drift out twice as slowly.

■ **Supplementary development of activity**

1 Move arms on the out breath only, let the movement accompany the breath.
2 Move whole body on the out breath as a physical warm-up.

■ **Additional outcomes**

Concentration on breath helps to focus the participants, particularly with a view to inner movement and vocal work.

BREATH 2

Aim: To enlarge vocalisation
Population: All
Conditions: Safety; not hurting
Time: 3 minutes
Equipment: None
Structure: Pairs

■ Activity

1 Partner, with flat of hand, repeatedly makes short, quick slaps on the other's back.
2 Other expels sounds of 'mmm', 'ah', etc.
3 Reverse roles.

■ Supplementary development of activity

Face partner and beat own chest with fists, expelling cries, opening mouth and throat so sound becomes louder.

BREATH 3

Aim: To encourage group to make sound
Population: All
Conditions: Some breath work in previous sessions
Time: 2 minutes
Equipment: None
Structure: Whole group

■ **Activity**

1 Whole group relax at knees and take in deep breath.
2 Very slowly, let out breath and make humming sound.
3 Allow sound to rise as eyes and arms lift to ceiling, until very loud.
4 Make movement shrink to floor; sound accompanies: sound and movement end simultaneously.

(Explain that some people may need more than one breath, and that they are able to breathe and make sound in own time.)

WARM-UP

BREATH 4

Aim: To introduce sound and breath together
Population: All
Conditions: None
Time: 2 minutes
Equipment: None
Structure: Whole group

■ **Activity**

1 Group can sit in circle.
2 All to breathe in through nose, make a huge yawn (no sound yet) and stretch arms.
3 Repeat with very slight sound.
4 Repeat noisily.
5 Divide group into three small groups; first group begins the yawn, second develops it, third finishes it, building up the sound per group.

■ **Supplementary development of activity**

1 Repeat above, but with a sigh and any accompanying movement.
2 Make sigh longer and more noisy each time.

GENERAL SPACE

Aims: Imitation skills, getting to know the environment
Population: All
Conditions: First session
Time: 4–5 minutes
Equipment: Choice of music
Structure: Individual, pairs, small groups

■ Activity

1 Individually the group move around the room, becoming familiar with the spaces, e.g. corners, centre of the room, sides of the room.
2 Leader suggests they begin by walking slowly into and out of each space.
3 Next they jog through the space.
4 Finally they are encouraged to run into and out of the spaces.
5 Leader can suggest activities, for example jump when you feel you have left/arrived in a space, skip from/to each space, jog-walk, stop as you arrive to explore a space.
6 Ensure changes of speed and direction during activity.
7 In pairs. Partner A leads B through part of the previous journey, exploring the spaces in the room. Partner remains behind/beside and follows the movement activity exactly. Change leader.
8 Repeat the above in a small group, changing leader at leader's suggestion.

■ Supplementary development of activity

1 Partners explore space as above with one leading and other following. Include gestures with hands as you go.
2 Change roles of leader and follower in own time without interrupting flow of movement.
3 Group leader moves and group follow.

■ Additional outcomes

1 Turn-taking and experience of exploring space in room.
2 Confidence in own movement and the space for moving through.

STRETCH 1

Aims: To identify and move body parts and muscle groups
Population: All
Conditions: Each session
Time: 5 minutes
Equipment: Music or percussion
Structure: Individual, partners

■ Activity

1 Leader verbally identifies body parts in turn, and encourages a gradual stretch and release for each named part.
2 Change the levels for stretching, e.g. lying, sitting, standing.
3 Use accompaniment if desired.

■ Supplementary development of activity

Partner B stretches A's limbs gently while lying on floor.

■ Additional outcomes

Awareness of sensation and articulation in body.

See *p. 298 for this activity used in another stage.*

STRETCH 2

Aim: To warm body for later physical work
Population: All
Conditions: None
Time: 15 minutes
Equipment: Music
Structure: Pairs

■ **Activity**

1 In pairs, stretch and relax a named body part in turn. Partner to echo.
2 Change energy level as progress is made through the body (i.e. begin very slowly). Leader could suggest they all move twice as slowly for the first 5–10 minutes.

■ **Additional outcomes**

Explore some new movements.

MASSAGE

Aims: To warm self and group; relaxation of muscles after physical exertion
Population: All
Conditions: None
Time: 5–10 minutes
Equipment: None
Structure: Whole group

■ Activity

1 Make a close circle, sitting or standing; one behind gently massages the shoulders of one in front.
2 Turn around and repeat.
3 Each to give feedback on how soft/hard they want massage.

See pp. 270 and 297 for this activity used in another stage.

WARM-UP

RELATIONSHIP 1

Aim: Initiating contact
Population: All
Conditions: None
Time: 2–5 minutes (depending on number in group)
Equipment: Bean bags or soft ball
Structure: Whole group

■ Activity

1 Throw the bean bag gently to someone and say their name. They catch it and throw it to a different person, again saying their name, and so on.
2 Each person to have a turn at throwing. Can throw to same person more than once.
3 Repeat and say something about the person as bean bag is thrown.

■ Additional outcomes

Giving feedback.

RELATIONSHIP 2

Aims: To notice others' movements and imitate in own body

Population: All

Conditions: None

Time: Variable (1–4 minutes)

Equipment: None

Structure: Whole group

■ Activity

1   In a circle one behind other, pass on the movement (given by leader). One behind copies the one in front. Let different movements emerge from the first one.

2   Repeat for 2–3 minutes, depending on the group's attention span.

PERSONAL SPACE 1

Aims: Impulse control and giving attention
Population: All
Conditions: None
Time: 4–5 minutes
Equipment: Music
Structure: Pairs

■ Activity

1 Find and face a partner, sitting.
2 Decide who will be initiator and who the follower.
3 The initiator explores slowly the space immediately in front and between the pair. They make shapes such as squares, circles and other pathways with their open hands through the air.
4 The partner follows, with their hands in a mirroring action.
5 At suggestion from leader they change roles several times while continuing to move.
6 Next the leader suggests they flow in and out of initiator and follower without stopping the movement, giving verbal hints as to when.
7 Repeat alone, giving non-verbal hints as to when.
8 Repeat without any hints.

■ Supplementary development of activity

1 Change from sitting to kneeling and repeat above.
2 Change to standing or travelling and repeat.
3 Use other parts of the body, own choice or as suggested by leader, for initiating and mirroring movement.
4 Encourage physical contact between partners.

■ Additional outcomes

Turn-taking followed by a feeling of co-operation between partners as they learn to give and take as one.

RHYTHM 1

Aim: To create a structure for group
Population: All
Conditions: None
Time: 5–6 minutes
Equipment: None
Structure: Whole group

■ Activity

1   Sitting in circle, leader claps out a simple rhythm and group copy.
2   Repeat with a more complex rhythm.
3   Volunteers take turns clapping out rhythm, group copy.

RHYTHM 2

Aim: To learn names
Population: All
Conditions: First meeting
Time: 5–10 minutes
Equipment: None
Structure: Whole group

■ **Activity**

1   Sitting in a circle, leader claps out a simple rhythm e.g. clap, clap, then says name.
2   Suggests whole group clap, clap and say names in interval between claps in turn around circle.
3   Repeat and reverse way round circle.

RHYTHM 3

Aim: To learn names
Population: All
Conditions: First session
Time: 5–10 minutes
Equipment: None
Structure: Whole group

■ Activity

1 Sitting down in a circle, leader starts by saying own name, accompanied by claps for the number of syllables in the name.
2 Leader suggests whole group copies the clapping of each name three times as participants clap their own names out around the circle.

RHYTHM 4

Aim: To learn names
Population: All
Conditions: Early session
Time: 5 minutes
Equipment: None
Structure: Whole group

■ Activity

1   Whole group sitting in a circle. Leader asks for suggestions for body sounds (non-vocal, such as clapping) from the group.
2   When three sounds have been suggested the leader puts them together to form a rhythm.
3   Group makes the rhythm and leader says their name in one of the intervals during it.
4   Whole group then continues with the rhythm, a name being said each time around the circle in turn at each repetition of the rhythm.
5   Repeat rhythm twice per person with group also saying name of each participant.
6   Repeat once per person—whole group says each name.

BODY CONTROL 3

Aim: To move whole body
Population: All
Conditions: None
Time: 5–10 minutes
Equipment: Music
Structure: Individual, partners

■ Activity

1 Curl and stretch whole body.
2 Sway whole body.
3 Leap and jump with feet together and apart.
4 In partners, move with whole body activity to music. When music stops, one makes a shape, other copies.
5 Reverse roles.

BALANCE 3

Aim: To follow gross motor pattern of another (see Section 2), sustained movement quality
Population: All
Conditions: None
Time: 5–8 minutes
Equipment: Slow music
Structure: Pairs, small groups, large group

■ Activity

1 Each person leads group in turn with a variety of balances.
2 Change balance on direction from group leader.
3 Repeat with a partner leading, changing balances in own time.
4 Followers to copy exactly the positions of stillness of partner.
5 Repeat as small then as large group, one balance then change leader.

■ Supplementary development of activity

1 Same as above but travel between each balance in own pattern.
2 Balance as a pair/small group/large group after travelling (in physical contact).

■ Additional outcomes

Containment of energy with others.
Leadership and following skills.
Creation of own movement forms and awareness of others.
Working with music as an accompaniment.

BALANCE 4

Aims: To promote body/self control; to create own movement structure; to integrate something new into own structure
Population: All
Conditions: Must be well warmed-up
Time: 5–6 minutes
Equipment: Music if required (rhythmical)
Structure: Individual, pairs

■ Activity

1 Hopping/jumping on the spot.
2 Change direction so as to travel forwards/backwards/sideways.
3 Make up own sequence of movement, exploring directions (e.g. two in each direction).

■ Supplementary development of activity

1 After own sequence created, share with a partner, teach it.
2 Return to own space and use one or two of the movements just learned from partner and find place for them in your sequence.
3 Show partner finished sequence; partner to identify which part had been theirs.

■ Additional outcomes

1 Can promote high energy in group.
2 Integration of a new movement into own pattern.
3 Awareness of how one movement can extend into different directions in space.
4 Sharing of movement.

BALANCE 1

Aims: To develop self-control and body awareness
Population: All
Conditions: None
Time: 4–5 minutes
Equipment: Music if desired
Structure: Individually and large group

■ **Activity**

1 On spot in circle, move one isolated body part (for example, circling an arm). Leader begins by modelling movement.
2 After a few of these, give opportunity for participants to identify and articulate one body part in turn around the group. Say out loud the name of the body part and the type of articulation.

■ **Supplementary development of activity**

1 Move two body parts.
2 Move one body part while rest of the body is in a specified shape, e.g. kneeling, sitting, legs astride.

■ **Additional outcomes**

1 Awareness in large group; turn-taking and following in rhythmic pattern.
2 Identification and articulation of body parts.

See p.108 for this activity used in another stage.

BALANCE 5

Aim: To reduce impulsivity
Population: All
Conditions: Adolescents may find blindfold more difficult
Time: 4–5 minutes
Equipment: Music, blindfold
Structure: Individually

■ Activity

1 As in the game of 'statues', move with the music and freeze in a balance when it stops.
2 Leader identifies balance at first, e.g. with one leg stretched behind.
3 Ask for a volunteer to 'stop' the music (with their back to the group).
4 Change volunteers.
5 After several turns, each member to create own balance.
6 On the 'stop', each member holds balance for 5 seconds, looks around and selects a balance from group for their next choice of balance.

■ Supplementary development of activity

Repeat 1–4 blindfolded.

■ Additional outcomes

1 Grounds (see Glossary) group and focuses them on centring (see Glossary) themselves.
2 Awareness of own and others' creativity.
3 Control of self and others (especially music operator).

See p. 225 for this activity used in another stage.

BALANCE 6

Aims: Conforming to structure; assertion; fun
Population: All
Conditions: Reinforce ground rules of safety; no tickling or violence
Time: 20 seconds per shape; 10 minutes total
Equipment: None
Structure: Pairs

■ Activity

1 In pairs, find own space, e.g. on a mat.
2 Both warm up by walking on hands and feet in own space.
3 When feel comfortable in shape, freeze in it strongly.
4 Partner A then attempts to unbalance their partner B from their shape; partner A can organise their energies in whatever way is best for unbalancing their partner.
5 Ensure both partners remain in specified shape for whole 20 seconds.

■ Supplementary development of activity

1 Repeat 1–5 with another specified shape.
2 Repeat 1–5 while both squatting and jumping (remain in identified space).

■ Additional outcomes

1 Contact via touch engendered.
2 Tolerance of frustration.
3 Awareness of own power stemming from body control and strength.

BALANCE 2

Aims: To develop control of body; to break 'rules'
Population: Children, adolescents, 'acting-out' adults
Conditions: Early sessions
Time: 5 minutes
Equipment: Drum
Structure: Individual

■ **Activity**

1 Group at one side of room.
2 Walk across room and stop very still when hear drum, which beats rhythmically. Aim is to continue walking, beginning wherever they like, while drum still playing. Since the overt rule is to 'stay still until the drum stops', they must aim to break that rule. Leader to ensure they understand that the rule can be broken.
3 Hold stillness while drum continues.
4 Ask for volunteer to drum. They can make a guess at who will break the rule each time.

■ **Supplementary development of activity**

1 Repeat, but run across room.
2 Repeat, but slide on belly across room.
3 Leader turns back on the group while drumming, so cannot see group.

■ **Additional outcomes**

Acknowledgement that 'rule-breaking' is possible in this structure.

See p.109 for this activity used in another stage.

LINES 1

Aim: To introduce concept of moving in space within a non-threatening structure
Population: All
Conditions: Early sessions
Time: 10 minutes
Equipment: Music—very slow, mystical
Structure: Individually

■ Activity

1 Imagine a line drawing you out into space; draw it invisibly with your hand. Stretch out along it and back towards your centre.
2 Use all the directions, carve shapes in the air with this line.
3 Now use the surfaces of the body and other limbs to describe these shapes, exploring all the possibilities.

■ Supplementary development of activity

1 In pairs, explore the qualities of your lines as one leads and the other follows (mirroring).
2 Perhaps give them some suggestions for lines, e.g. short/long, curved/straight, continuous flow/interrupted flow, high/low.
3 Change leader.
4 Show the group some lines you have made on a large sheet of paper and have them all move whole body to each of these.

■ Additional outcomes

An awareness of their own and others' creativity.

RELATIONSHIP 3

Aims: To initiate, maintain and leave a relationship
Population: All
Conditions: None
Time: 3–5 minutes
Equipment: None
Structure: Pairs

■ Activity

1 In pairs, one initiates slowly making contact with the other's hands to encourage swaying. Maintain contact, then say goodbye.
2 Change initiator; this time focus on a different body part, for example feet or shoulders.
3 Both partners say goodbye and leave each other by moving away into a new space alone.

■ Supplementary development of activity

1 Repeat 1–3 above and after leaving partner make contact with another person.
2 Repeat 1–3 with that person.

■ Additional outcomes

Receiving and gaining attention.

RELATIONSHIP 4

Aim: To assert an effect on the group
Population: All
Conditions: None
Time: 4–5 minutes
Equipment: Possibly music, if group lacking in confidence
Structure: Whole group

■ Activity

1 In a circle, session leader leads the group in a 'do as I do' dance. Vary the speed, strength and body part.
2 In a line, repeat step 1.
3 Travelling in a line, repeat step 1.
4 Session leader could suggest changes in leadership or allow group to decide. Change leaders frequently (every 30–40 seconds).

QUALITY 1

Aim: To develop quality of strength
Population: All
Conditions: None
Time: 2–5 minutes
Equipment: Drum
Structure: Individual

■ Activity

1 Leader suggests group imagine they are moving like a tiger stalking its prey.
2 On the sound of the drum they pounce on the prey.
3 Group gather strength to sound of drum then release it strongly in pouncing movement.

QUALITY 2

Aim: To develop quality of strength
Population: Adolescents
Conditions: Safety ground rule
Time: 2–5 minutes
Equipment: Possibly tambourine
Structure: Individual

■ Activity

Leader involves group in rehearsing 'kung fu'-like actions with arms and legs, encouraging jumping, kicking and turning.

■ Supplementary development of activity

1   Remain on own mat.
2   Jump to the next mat with a 'kung fu' action.

QUALITY 3

Aim: To develop quality of lightness
Population: All
Conditions: None
Time: 2–5 minutes
Equipment: None
Structure: Individual

■ Activity

1 Leader suggests group move as though a feather falling gently in the breeze.
2 Encourage circling, swaying, falling and floating movements in a quiet atmosphere.

■ Supplementary development of activity

1 Only using hands and arms.
2 Only using feet and legs.

QUALITY 4

Aim: To introduce quality of suddenness
Population: All
Conditions: None
Time: 2–3 minutes
Equipment: None
Structure: Pairs

■ Activity

1 Leader suggests labelling selves A and B.
2 Partner A then attempts to startle partner B by jumping, clapping and saying 'boo'. Partner ignores them.
3 Reverse roles.

■ Additional outcomes

Learning not to respond to provocation.

QUALITY 5

Aim: To introduce quality of suddenness
Population: Children, adolescents
Conditions: None
Time: 2 minutes
Equipment: Drum
Structure: Individual

■ **Activity**

1 Leader suggests they move as though being shocked by a repeated loud noise when drum sounds.
2 Encourage movement and stillness alternately.

QUALITY 6

Aim: To introduce sustained movement
Population: All
Conditions: None
Time: 2–3 minutes
Equipment: None
Structure: Pairs

■ **Activity**

1 Leader suggests partner A moves arm in a gesture towards partner B.
2 Now make the same gesture at half the speed. Partner B watches intently as the gesture is made.
3 Now halve the speed again. Partner B gives feedback as to whether it seemed slower.
4 Finally, halve the speed again.
5 Reverse roles.

■ **Additional outcomes**

Focusing of attention.

BREATH 5

Aim: To energise, and facilitate 'letting go'
Population: All
Conditions: Warmed up
Time: 1 minute
Equipment: None
Structure: Whole group

■ **Activity**

1 Group in circle. Using elbows alternately, punch backwards, breathing out at same time.
2 Make a sound as breathe out.

PAIRS RESISTANCE 1

Aim: To introduce idea of going with as well as against another's resistance
Population: Adults, adolescents
Conditions: None
Time: 3–4 minutes
Equipment: None
Structure: Partners

■ Activity

1 Find a partner; one stands behind the other, who is kneeling. Both face the front.
2 Make contact with hands.
3 Resist and go with partner's resistance alternately.
4 Ensure eyes are closed throughout activity.
5 The movement maintains an up-down direction as each partner flows in and out of their resistance.
6 Leader times the activity carefully, suggests change in roles.

■ Supplementary development of activity

1 Facing partner, hand-to-hand contact, repeat 1–5 above.
2 Discussion with partner on theme of resisting, contact, etc.
3 Discussion with partner on what liked/disliked about interaction.

■ Additional outcomes

1 Awareness of how participants individually contribute to or go with resistance from another.
2 How others affect our need to resist or flow with the direction of the resistance.

PAIRS RESISTANCE 2

Aim: To encourage personal strength
Population: All
Conditions: Repeat safety ground rules. First few sessions
Time: 10–15 minutes
Equipment: None
Structure: Pairs

■ Activity

1 Partners sit back to back (backs in contact and knees bent) and, as leader counts aloud from 1 to 10, they push each other towards the other side of the room with all the strength they can muster.
2 Change partners, this time standing and shoulder to shoulder (side to side).
3 Repeat pushing game with leader counting again and with other shoulders in contact.
4 Change partners again, this time hips to hips.
5 Change partners, hands to hands.
6 Change partners, hands to shoulders (making eye contact throughout).

■ Supplementary development of activity

Could add a line between partners for them to attempt to push each other across.

■ Additional outcomes

1 Should have 'resisted' almost every member of group by end of activity.
2 Having begun with the safer relationship (back to back) the group finish with a more open relationship (making eye contact and facing partner).

PERSONAL SPACE 2

Aim: Reaching through and receiving another in personal space

Population: Adults

Conditions: Some eye contact required, when group has become somewhat cohesive

Time: 4–5 minutes

Equipment: None

Structure: Large group

■ Activity

1 Find a partner you feel you know and like. Number as 1 and 2.
2 1s make an outer circle around inner circle of 2s. Face partners and make eye contact.
3 Inner circle only, smile and reach with hands to receive contact with partner's hands.
4 Outer circle partners respond with smile and give hand contact.
5 Inner circle only, move round to the next person on right and repeat.
6 Continue to move round to right until returned to original partner.
7 Change inner and outer circles. Repeat with new people in the inner circle initiating contact.
8 Discussion in partners of any difficulties; what was the best thing about it, what did it remind you of?

■ Supplementary development of activity

1 Repeat with a verbal greeting or name.
2 Repeat with eyes closed. Leader could ensure people unaware of who they were facing, that both reach out at the same time or give a choice, and give a longer time for hand contact with one or two participants only. Awareness could be stimulated by leader asking

questions such as, 'can you tell if this person is male, female, outgoing, reticent?', etc.

■ Additional outcomes

Members become more sensitive to each other and how they feel when people enter their personal space.

PERSONAL SPACE 3

Aim: To explore personal space
Population: Children, adults
Conditions: None
Time: 3 minutes
Equipment: Possibly music
Structure: Individual

■ **Activity**

1   Leader suggests that participants imagine they are trapped in a net of some kind. Their task is to find a way out, but one part of their body (either given by the leader or their own choice) remains fixed to the floor throughout.

2   They are encouraged to imagine exploring the net to find a hole big enough to climb out through.

■ **Supplementary development of activity**

1   Imagine another material enclosure on edge of personal space. Only by their reaching to furthest points around body does it become manifested.

2   Somewhere there is a gap in the enclosure through which to crawl. Leader could suggest the texture of the enclosure as being soft, glass, plastic, etc. Again emphasis is on the exploration around the body into the space immediately surrounding the participant, as far as they can reach while one part of the body is fixed to the wall/floor.

■ **Additional outcomes**

Heightened awareness of the movement opportunities within their own space.

PERSONAL SPACE 4 (SHADOW BOXING)

Aim: To co-operate in a movement dialogue, taking turns
Population: Adolescents
Conditions: Reinforce safety rules
Time: 3 minutes
Equipment: None
Structure: Pairs, one behind and slightly to side of other

■ Activity

1 Name of movement game is 'shadow boxing'; in pairs, A and B stand one behind the other.
2 A initiates a movement and freezes in a final shape, waits for B to imitate exactly.
3 A moves again, B imitates.
4 They turn to face the other way, this time B initiates.
5 Repeat for several turns.

■ Supplementary development of activity

1 Make two or three movements each time but in slow motion.
2 Repeat exercise in a group of three.

■ Additional outcomes

Some control of movement impulse and active management of waiting in turn-taking.

PERSONAL SPACE 5
(SPACE ACTION DANCES)

Aims: To develop anticipation and prediction skills; awareness of the body in space

Population: Children and adolescents

Conditions: None

Time: 5–10 minutes

Equipment: None

Structure: Large group and pairs

■ Activity

1 Name of activity is 'space action dances' (see Section 2 'Laban movement analysis'). Start with large group sitting in a circle.
2 Leader moves arms, with an appropriate song, in the spatial planes, i.e. rocking side to side, up and down, forward and back, and all the way round.
3 Whole group sing and copy movements in rhythm.
4 Divide into pairs and move the dance together; change it in any way.
5 Share dance in fours when completed.

■ Supplementary development of activity

1 Could involve more of body, e.g. spin round on seat for 'all the way round'.
2 Practice sideways rolling in pairs or individually.
3 Forward/backward rolls individually on mats or from behind over partner or leader's back. The leader sits with legs astride catching roller as they bend over one shoulder and put hands on floor, curling in at waist, their head being protected as they are helped into and out of forward roll.
4 Spin around with partner, spin each other.
5 Jump with a partner, over a partner; in a group of three, two outsiders support and help the middle one from

a low position to jump high off the ground and land back softly with knees bent.

6 Partners, when they have practised the above exercises, could choose three favourites and put them together so they flow one to the other.

■ Additional outcomes

Awareness of spatial directions. Experience of body activities with the focus on which direction they move through.

SHAPES 1

Aims: To move and be still in group shaping
Population: Adolescents, adults
Conditions: None
Time: 5 minutes
Equipment: Could use music or percussion
Structure: Threes

■ Activity

1   Label the three members A, B and C. A initiates by moving slowly and smoothly into a shape; B follows and fits with that shape, then C moves to fit with that shape. Hold shape for a few seconds.
2   Repeat the above with B leading, then C; thus members take turns to initiate, yet the group form a unified whole.
3   Discuss:
    (a)   what you noticed
    (b)   how you initiated
    (c)   how you maintained the relationship.
    (d)   Is this a recognisable pattern?

■ Supplementary development of activity

1   Repeat steps 1 and 2 above but this time with the As finding another group's A, meeting up and relating to them. The Bs and Cs stay attached, as though append-ages, to their group's A, supporting the shape initiated.
2   Repeat step 1 above but this time the two As find another two As from another group and relate to them. Bs and Cs stay supporting their own group's shape.
3   Repeat above until all As in the group are relating/inter-acting (non-verbally) with their supporters (Bs and Cs).

■ Additional outcomes

1 An awareness of feeling unique, yet conforming to the group.
2 Acknowledgement of and support for the uniqueness of self.
3 An improvised choreography, which the group maintains.

See p. 207 for this activity used in another stage.

WHISPERS

Aim: To practice imitation skills
Population: Adolescents, adults
Conditions: None
Time: 5 minutes
Equipment: None
Structure: Whole group or several small groups

■ **Activity**

1 Group in circle standing one behind the other.
2 Leader gives instructions that each person should imitate any movement, however slight, that they notice the person in front making. No one, however, is to move purposefully, other than to imitate the person in front.
3 The leader makes one purposeful movement to begin the group movement. The person behind the leader repeats it so that the movement is passed around the circle.
4 Allow group to experience the movements that evolve from all the unconscious movement emitted from members.

■ **Additional outcomes**

Awareness of how much movement we generate without full consciousness.

See p. 235 and 300 for this activity used in another stage.

OBJECTS

Aims: To make an effect on the environment; to relate to an object; to work with anger

Population: All

Conditions: Early sessions, safety aspects reinforced

Time: 5–10 minutes

Equipment: Soft ball, football, netball, large table, chair

Structure: Individual, pairs

■ Activity

1 After reinforcing safety aspects, give each member the opportunity to throw the ball against the wall.
2 Ensure an adequate distance away from the wall, give plenty of space between people. Begin with gentle throw developing into a strong, hard throw with all energy.
3 Regulate how they are to retrieve the ball.
4 What sound goes with the strong throw? All to make this at once.
5 What movement feels the most satisfying to make the throw?
6 In pairs, one to throw, the other to observe and retrieve ball. Encourage use of whole body, discuss in pairs what name might accompany the throw (someone from your life).
7 Share name in large group.

■ Supplementary development of activity

1 Push or pull a large heavy object (e.g. someone sitting on a chair, a table that is being pushed by others against the participant). Do this for a limited time period, e.g. 20 seconds.
2 Discuss in pairs where/when this type of energy is used in each life and what happens next.

3 In turn, enact the scenario, beginning with the pushing and ending with own ending; use sound and words where they arise spontaneously.

4 Partner then moves the scenario in exactly the same way to show their partner a mirror of their movement story.

5 5 minutes to explore a different ending for self.

6 Enact new ending.

7 Discuss with partner how the exercise gave an understanding of patterns in our lives and to what extent learning about different use of self took place.

■ Additional outcomes

1 Acknowledgement of anger.

2 Recognition of a tension-provoking person in life and the patterns used to deal with frustration.

3 Some insight into the effect they can make on others with their use of energy.

BRIDGES

Aim: To introduce contact
Population: All
Conditions: Not to be used if little body control
Time: 10–15 minutes
Equipment: None
Structure: Pairs, small groups

■ Activity

1 One partner makes a bridge shape.
2 Partner moves under the bridge without touching it.
3 Any touch noticed by the bridge can result in them making a 'buzz' sound.
4 Change roles.
5 Repeat; this time touch is allowed.
6 Repeat with three different shapes.

■ Supplementary development of activity

1 Partner to go over the bridge instead of under.
2 Groups of three or four make an 'over-under' shape together and volunteer moves through without/with touch. Repeat with new shape and new volunteer.

■ Additional outcomes

1 Making physical contact without it predominating.
2 Development of trust.
3 Beginning to work on separation and merging with another.

IMAGERY

Aims: To engage with an image through movement; to stimulate the imagination; to encourage spontaneous movement

Population: All

Conditions: None

Time: 15–20 minutes

Equipment: Leader prepares drawn/written images on small pieces of paper

Structure: Individual, small groups

■ Activity

1 Leader draws an image and shows it to the group, who then respond to it in movement for 20 seconds or so.
2 Leader folds up pieces of paper with drawn/written images upon them; each member selects one, then for 2 minutes explores the image in movement.
3 Repeat step 2.
4 With a partner, try to guess the image from the movement responses.
5 Now each partner gives an image in turn for partner to respond to for 20 seconds. The image is given verbally, e.g. 'move like a lion sneaking up on a deer'.

■ Supplementary development of activity

1 In small groups, the leader secretly gives a visual or verbal image to each group.
2 Each group spends 4 minutes preparing to respond.
3 Each group shares their response with the whole group who may guess the image given.

■ Additional outcomes

Development of symbolic expression, use of expressive movement in communication, development of a specific theme which the group is addressing, introduction of a relevant theme for the group.

See p. 223 for this activity used in another stage.

BODY BOUNDARY 2

Aims: Centring (see Glossary), self-assertion
Population: All
Conditions: None
Time: 15 minutes
Equipment: None
Structure: Partners

■ **Activity**

1 Contract body inwards and hold tightly.
2 Partner tries to open up, but stay tightly closed. (Give a limited time for this, e.g. 20 seconds, and state that there should be no violence or tickling.)
3 Change roles.
4 Offer a short discussion time on the issue of being closed off/someone wanting you to open up.

■ **Supplementary development of activity**

1 Using fists only, partner this time attempts to open up the fist.
2 Both have eyes closed.

■ **Additional outcomes**

1 Awareness of own strength and the development of a relationship with another group member.
2 Acknowledgement of need to remain closed at times.

BODY BOUNDARY 3

Aims: To give and receive peer attention; to develop trust, sensitivity and awareness of self affecting others

Population: Adolescents, adults

Conditions: Safety rules

Time: 10 minutes

Equipment: None

Structure: Pairs, whole group

■ Activity

1 All stand in a circle.
2 Pummel all soft areas of own body and chest (making sound).
3 Pair up, one partner pummels with loose fists the other's calves, thighs, buttocks, backs, shoulders, upper arms.
4 Finish by stroking from the top of their head down to their feet slowly in one gentle sweep.
5 Repeat with a new partner (i.e. person on other side of you in the circle).
6 Notice the difference in contact between the two people who have massaged you. Notice your responses to them and any differences.

■ Supplementary development of activity

1 After the above, open up a large group discussion that encourages each person to give feedback to those who massaged them.
2 Ask how it felt to be getting and giving this kind of attention from each other.

■ Additional outcomes

1 A recognition of the part physical contact plays in their lives.

2 A new level of relationship with peers.
3 The ability to give and receive feedback from peers.
4 Giving and receiving attention in a group.

See p. 270 for this activity used in another stage.

BODY BOUNDARY 4

Aim: Differentiation of self from environment
Population: Adolescents, adults
Conditions: None
Time: 10 minutes
Equipment: None
Structure: Individual

■ Activity

1 Lying on the floor. Move so that all the skin areas of your body come into contact with the floor.
2 Turn over and repeat.
3 Do not miss any areas, give them all a massage.

■ Supplementary development of activity

1 Continue moving in contact with the floor but now with only your large muscles.
2 Move from one muscle group to another, exploring the balance as you go.
3 Now focus on the bones only.
4 Move so that joints and bones make contact with the floor; again balance as you go.

■ Additional outcomes

1 Awareness of the periphery of the body through to the inner aspects of the body.
2 Experience in stillness as balancing is worked with.
3 Establishment of the floor as a friend and supporter.

BODY BOUNDARY 5

Aims: Differentiation of self from the environment, body awareness
Population: Adults
Conditions: None
Time: 10 minutes
Equipment: Gentle music
Structure: Individual

■ Activity

1 Participants lie on the floor, keeping their eyes closed throughout the activity; they imagine they are floating in water, or through the air, their limbs gently supported.
2 Slowly move limbs, beginning with arms.
3 Carve a way through air or water and rise up to a standing position.
4 Begin to walk; carve shapes with limbs as travel through space.

■ Supplementary development of activity

1 Imagine being in a different substance, such as glue, honey or sand, carving shapes through it with arms, legs, body, head.
2 Repeat the activity with eyes open.
3 Use different sequences, for example, from standing to travelling to lying.

■ Additional outcomes

1 Giving a sense of restrained flow.
2 Assertion of a clear air pattern through space.
3 Experiencing body boundaries and tension patterns.

FLOOR PATTERN 3

Aim: To say goodbye
Population: All
Conditions: End of session or period of treatment, or if
a group member/leader is leaving
Time: 10–15 minutes
Equipment: Hoops or mats perhaps
Structure: Individual

■ Activity

1 Make a straight, direct pathway toward one specific space in the room. Scan the room first and select somewhere.
2 Repeat, moving from space to space or object to object.
3 Repeat, moving from person to person.
4 Repeat all of the above, but interacting non-verbally before leaving for next object/space/person.
5 Notice how long interaction takes and whether you initiate, maintain, respond or ignore interaction play. How do you leave?
6 Discuss in whole group:
   (a) how participants were left,
   (b) how they left others, spaces, objects.
Notice any patterns/differences between people/objects/spaces. Relate to 'leaving' theme.

■ Additional outcomes

Awareness of how leaving or being left can affect individuals and group.

LEVEL 2

Aims: To promote adaptability in movement and stillness between levels in space

Population: Children

Conditions: None

Time: 3 minutes

Equipment: Percussion if required

Structure: Individual

■ Activity

1 Make a high shape and hold it before spiralling down to the floor, sinking slowly into it as you arrive.
2 Explore spirals from high to low and low to high.
3 Make stops at three different places on the spiral.
4 Make two stops on the way up the spiral and three stops on the way down. Choice of how long these stops take.

■ Supplementary development of activity

1 Vary the speed of the spiral so as to experience stillness from sustained and sudden movement.
2 Ensure same/different shape in stillness each time.
3 Repeat all the above with a partner or in a threesome, complementing stillnesses.
4 Leader could direct the whole activity so that all participants are moving and stopping at one time.

■ Additional outcomes

Some decision-making skills used in choice of when and for how long to stop in stillness. Body control and extension of movement range.

LEVEL 3

Aims: To engender co-operation in small group; to encourage movement/experience in the high level
Population: Adolescents, adults
Conditions: Warmed up physically
Time: 2–3 minutes
Equipment: None
Structure: Threes

■ Activity

1 Groups of three, volunteer stands in middle, other two either side supporting the middle one under arms and at forearms/hands.
2 The two people on the outside assist the middle one to jump up; they begin and land with knees bent.
3 Repeat with new person in the middle.

■ Additional outcomes

1 Support of another.
2 Experience jumping with assistance.
3 Energising for whole group.

INTRODUCTION TO THEME

AIR PATTERN 1

Aim: To use an object as an extension of the self
Population: All
Conditions: None
Time: 4–5 minutes
Equipment: Pieces of fabric of various shapes, colours, sizes and weights
Structure: Individual

■ Activity

1 Each participant selects a piece of fabric.
2 Explore its properties by moving it in space, on the spot and travelling.
3 Use it to carve out shapes in the air while on the spot.
4 Use it to carve out shapes in the air while travelling and changing directions in space.

■ Supplementary development of activity

1 Move on the floor with the fabric.
2 Use it as a magic carpet and take a journey with it for 2 minutes.
3 Move with a partner and with fabric.
4 Using one very large piece of fabric work in fours or the whole group, with focus on moving with fabric.

BODY SHAPE

Aim: To develop awareness of the body shape in space
Population: Children
Conditions: None
Time: 4–5 minutes
Equipment: Possibly music/percussion
Structure: Individual, partners

■ **Activity**

Leader gives direction for all participants to make their bodies into a specific shape, for example:

(a) like a ball—as *round* as you can,
(b) like a wall—as *wide* as you can,
(c) like a lamppost—as *tall* as you can,
(d) like a giant—as *big* as you can,
(e) like a ladybird—as *small* as you can,
(f) like a twig—as *crooked* as you can.

■ **Supplementary development of activity**

1 Repeat (a)–(f) above in pairs. Encourage physical contact.
2 Give shapes to each pair, e.g. star, cross, spiral, letters.
3 Repeat step 2 above but in threes or fours, and ask them to spell out a simple name from the group (e.g. John).
4 Small group could move into any shape above, from e.g. walking, running, jumping, skipping, using music/percussion for travelling steps, then leader stopping it for groups to make shapes. Groups could see who got into specified shape first.

■ **Additional outcomes**

Emphasis on shapes such as pointed, angular, round, twisted, as an individual, in twos, and within a group.

DIRECTIONALITY 1

Aims: Movement imitation, turn-taking, giving of attention
Population: All
Conditions: None
Time: 5 minutes
Equipment: Music if desired
Structure: Small groups (4–5)

■ Activity

1 All standing in a line, one behind the other.
2 Leader of line moves one arm sideways and those behind copy at the same time.
3 Leader moves both arms and all copy.
4 Leader moves legs and/or arms for all to copy.
5 Change leader.

■ Supplementary development of activity

1 Leader travels, using only feet.
2 Whole group become one line (the small groups join up).

PIN ROLL

Aim: To be effective with others
Population: All
Conditions: Give enough space to each pair
Time: 10 minutes
Equipment: None (could make a 'goal' at one end for partner to roll towards)
Structure: Pairs

■ Activity

In pairs, roll partner along floor in a pin roll (arms stretched out above head). Use different body parts, such as feet, head, hands, to propel partner.

■ Supplementary development of activity

1 Could roll individually in pin rolls across the floor.
2 Hold hands with a partner and roll together.

BODY CONTROL 4

Aims: To be aware of movement and stillness
Population: All
Conditions: None
Time: 4–5 minutes
Equipment: Light classical music, if desired
Structure: Individual

■ **Activity**

1 Rhythm of walking and being still suggested; e.g. walk, walk, still, still.
2 Each participant makes own rhythm of being still and walking.

■ **Additional outcomes**

Development of internal control.

PRE-LATERALITY 1

Aim: Co-ordinate arms and legs in rhythm
Population: All
Conditions: None
Time: 5–8 minutes
Equipment: Marching music if desired, drums
Structure: Individually, whole group

■ Activity

1   Marching with same arms and legs, i.e. both right arm and leg move together then both left arm and leg.
2   Marching with opposite arms to legs (i.e. right arm with left leg—it may be better, though, not to mention right and left specifically).
3   March in whole group with different leaders.
4   Could incorporate drummers accompanying marchers.
5   Leader could clap out rhythm.

■ Supplementary development of activity

1   Create own phrase individually using arm/leg co-ordination and march it out around the room.
2   Half group share with other half and change over.

■ Additional outcomes

Development of awareness of the two sides of the body.

PRE-LATERALITY 2

Aim: Body awareness
Population: All
Conditions: None
Time: 5–6 minutes
Equipment: Ribbon, material
Structure: Individually, partners

■ Activity

1 Lying on back, move in co-ordination arms and legs, opening and closing; leader directs.
2 The partner who is lying watches the partner who is standing up in front of them and copies movement of arms and legs as though a mirror.
3 Leader may suggest shaking of one hand, kicking one leg, as well as two arms and/or two legs moving together.
4 Partner is only to use one side of body now—identify by tying material, ribbon, or giving something to hold.
5 Change roles.

■ Supplementary development of activity

1 Repeat 1–5 with both standing up facing each other.
2 Repeat 1–5 with one behind the other.
3 Repeat 1–5 with partners side by side.

■ Additional outcomes

Stress of one side of the body and then the other.

See p. 218 for this activity used in another stage.

FALLING

Aim: To develop sense of 'giving in' to gravity
Population: Adolescents, adults
Conditions: After some trust between participants established
Time: 4–5 minutes
Equipment: None
Structure: Whole group, partners

■ Activity

1 In a line, one in front of the other, close together. The second participant down the line (the catcher) places their arms around the first participant from behind.
2 The first participant then gently and slowly allows their ankles, knees and hips to collapse and they fall against their catcher. Catcher ensures they fall against them and slide down them to the floor.
3 The catcher takes as much weight from the faller as appropriate. Faller lets go into the floor.
4 The third participant (the next catcher) then moves forward and places themselves close to the body of the next faller (the previous catcher).
5 Repeat falling and catching until all in the line have fallen to the floor, and then the last one in the line turns around; the others stand up; and the whole activity is repeated, starting from the back of the line.

■ Supplementary development of activity

1 Partners can practice the roles of catcher and faller.
2 Discussion about being caught, letting go, falling and catching.

■ Additional outcomes

1 A 'letting go' of the physical and emotional self.
2 Trusting the self sufficiently to be safe in the arms of another.
3 Trusting self to catch, hold and take care of another.

AIR PATTERN 2

Aims: To identify self and make own shapes in air pattern
Population: Children
Conditions: None
Time: 2 minutes
Equipment: None
Structure: Individually

■ Activity

1   Each participant sitting down draws out letter shapes in the air as suggested by the leader.
2   Make the letter shapes bigger, use a larger area of space so you have to move.
3   Repeat, drawing out own name.
4   Repeat, drawing out another group member's name.
5   Repeat, drawing out one word.

■ Supplementary development of activity

Partner could guess the word/name.

AIR PATTERN 3

Aim: To encourage movement of limbs in space
Population: All
Conditions: None
Time: 4 minutes
Equipment: Possibly abstract music
Structure: Individual

■ **Activity**

1 All participants move in space, carving out shapes in the air with arms, then legs, then head only.
2 Repeat, co-ordinating limbs and other surfaces of body as you carve way through space.

■ **Additional outcomes**

1 Assert own movement in space.
2 Make an effect on the environment.

MASKS

Aim: To promote awareness of masks in life
Population: Adults, adolescents
Conditions: Once safety and trust are established in the group
Time: 40–60 minutes
Equipment: A variety of objects
Structure: Individual

■ Activity

1 Bring to the session a variety of objects provided by participants and/or leader.
2 Each participant makes a mask to go over face and/or head. Spend about 30 minutes on this.
3 Using the mask, explore sitting/kneeling/standing positions for this mask. If large mirrors are available have group face mirror for these explorations.
4 Next have group move in steps to a repetitive rhythm that is representative of the mask. If using mirrors have them face front all the time and move across space in front of mirror in turn.
5 Partners. Share an improvisation in turn where you use the positions and step pattern. Partner to watch and be aware of how it makes you feel.
6 Discuss what you felt as you observed your partner. What masks did you use? What are you hiding behind these?

■ Supplementary development of activity

Imagine drinking a potion that affects the body. Explore in mask how the potion makes participants move, e.g. cold, numb, heavy, rigid, frozen as though a stone.

■ Additional outcomes

An awareness of how masks can hide/reveal the inner self.

BREATH 6

Aims: To focus on in and out breath in movement
Population: Adults
Conditions: None
Time: 5–10 minutes
Equipment: Meditation or healing music
Structure: Whole group

■ **Activity**

1 Leader suggests group sit/lie in own space, eyes closed.
2 Focus on out breath, breathing out through nose and relaxing body several times, use evenly the whole of the chest and abdomen to expel air slowly.
3 Focus on in breath (through nose); slowly allow air to enter abdomen and chest region.
4 Focus on pause between in and out or out and in breaths. Be aware of what part of your breath cycle has the pause/still point.
5 Begin to move as an accompaniment to:
   (a) out breath,
   (b) in breath,
   (c) pause.
   Aim to rise to standing and travelling in own time.

■ **Supplementary development of activity**

Breathe out as though through toes and other areas of the body, e.g. backs. Imagine every cell of the body expanding as you exhale through the nose.

■ **Additional outcomes**

Inner focus encouraged, awareness of body in co-ordination and movement as an accompaniment of the breath.

TRUST 1

Aim: To develop trust in group
Population: All
Conditions: Early in sessions, safety rules emphasised
Time: 10–15 minutes
Equipment: None
Structure: Partners

■ Activity

1 Partners catch each other in turn but only when the 'faller' decides to fall against catcher.
2 Catcher is to ensure feet are on wide base, one behind the other and knees bent slightly; hands wide, ready to catch partner by shoulder blades as they fall backwards.
3 Faller to stand 15 to 25 centimetres away at first, then gradually extend distance of fall. Keep body rigid. Catcher simply catches and returns them to upright position.
4 Reverse roles.

■ Supplementary development of activity

Repeat above with faller falling towards partner, partner catches them by the front of their shoulders.

■ Additional outcomes

Trusting own weight to another.

BODY CONTROL 5

Aims: To promote awareness, rhythm and impulse control
Population: All
Conditions: None
Time: 3 minutes
Equipment: Strong, rhythmic music
Structure: Whole group

■ **Activity**

1 Group sit on floor and rock backwards and forwards, hands behind head.
2 The music is then played and group rock in time.
3 At several points leader stops music, when the group have to freeze in their positions.
4 Leader needs to vary the length of the pauses between playing the music.

RHYTHM 5

Aim: Imitation skills
Population: All
Conditions: None
Time: 5 minutes
Equipment: None
Structure: Partners

■ **Activity**

1 In partners, one gently taps out a simple rhythm on the back of the other, who then stamps/claps back the same rhythm.
2 Reverse roles.
3 Repeat with more complex rhythms.

RHYTHM 6

Aim: Awareness of inner rhythm
Population: All
Conditions: None
Time: 5 minutes
Equipment: A drum each
Structure: Whole group

■ **Activity**

1 Participants to engage in vigorous activity, then place hand on pulse/heart to feel the beat.
2 Drum out the rhythm.
3 Stamp out the rhythm.
4 Clap out the rhythm.

SHAPES AND WORDS

Aims: To explore emotions and associated postures in a group
Population: All
Conditions: None
Time: 5 minutes
Equipment: None
Structure: Threes

■ Activity

1 Leader says three words in turn that describe emotions (e.g. joy, fear, etc.).
2 For each word in turn, each group member takes a turn to make a shape in the centre of the circle. The other two members complement it, so that the whole group shape represents the emotion.
3 Leader indicates when each member is to take up the shape by saying '1, 2, 3' for each word.

ROCK

Aim: To hold own ground
Population: All
Conditions: No violence
Time: 2 minutes
Equipment: None
Structure: Pairs

■ Activity

1 For one member of each pair, leader says 'make your-self like a rock'. Encourage use of wide base, low to the floor.
2 Partner attempts to push them over.
3 Change over.

■ Supplementary development of activity

Do with several partners.

■ Additional outcomes

1 Self-assertion.
2 Development of the quality of strength with bound flow (see Section 2, 'Laban movement analysis').

LOCOMOTION 4

Aims: To move in accordance with a set rhythm, travelling (see Glossary) in a co-ordinated, rhythmic experience
Population: Children, adults
Conditions: None
Time: 10 minutes
Equipment: Drum, music of your choice
Structure: Whole group as individuals, in partners, threes

■ Activity

1 Leader beats out a rhythm on the drum or puts on the music.
2 Leader varies the rhythm and calls out ways of travelling (e.g. walk, gallop, slide, jump, slither).

■ Supplementary development of activity

1 Join up with a partner and follow the pattern of travelling the partner selects, while leader continues to beat out a rhythm; then repeat, reversing roles.
2 Repeat in threes, small groups, periodically changing the person deciding the pattern.
3 Let a volunteer beat out rhythm on drum or select the music for the group.

■ Additional outcomes

1 More trust develops as the leader is accepted.
2 All members can initiate their own ideas for travelling within the safety of a clear rhythmic pattern.
3 The group learns to follow the lead from others and turn-taking is experienced in taking the lead.

See p.110 for this activity used in another stage.

LOCOMOTION 5

Aim: To encourage forms of locomotion
Population: All
Conditions: None
Time: 5–10 minutes
Equipment: None
Structure: Whole group

■ Activity

1 Leader suggests group walk around space in readiness for a movement activity suggested by a volunteer.
2 At any point in time a participant (selected by leader or self-selected) can call out a travelling activity (e.g. hop, jump, roll, etc.).
3 The group continue the specified activity until another volunteer participant calls out an activity, at which point the group moves in that manner.
4 Repeat so that all members have been 'caller volunteers', whether spontaneously or at direction of leader.

(There is no need for 'callers' to drop out of the group's movement.)

■ Additional outcomes

Participants have opportunity to lead group.

SHAPES 2

Aims: To explore characteristics and/or emotions associated with postures in a group

Population: All
Conditions: None
Time: 10–15 minutes
Equipment: None
Structures: Threes or fours

■ **Activity**

1 In turn each member (the initiator) takes up a shape in the centre that expresses how they feel, or one unique characteristic of themselves.
2 Rest of the group silently ask themselves: What is being expressed? Does this person need physical support? Distance? Touch?
3 Then each group member chooses to enter that space or not. Once they have entered they respond to the person's shape with another; they may add to it as seems appropriate, then leave.
4 The initiator returns to the group when they feel there have been enough responses.
5 Group ask what was especially satisfying. Initiator asks group what they thought he/she was communicating to them. Initiator tells group how he/she felt they responded. Group ask themselves what their role was (e.g. support, self-interest, etc.).

■ **Supplementary development of activity**

Repeat in whole group, using centre of circle for each to enter in turn.

■ Additional outcomes

1 To be part of a group yet separate from it.
2 Expression of 'differentness', and that being accepted.

SHAPES 1

Aims: To move and be still in group shaping
Population: Adolescents, adults
Conditions: None
Time: 5 minutes
Equipment: Could use music or percussion
Structure: Threes

■ Activity

1   Label the three members A, B and C. A initiates by moving slowly and smoothly into a shape; B follows and fits with that shape, then C moves to fit with that shape. Hold shape for a few seconds.
2   Repeat the above with B leading, then C; thus members take turns to initiate, yet the group form a unified whole.
3   Discuss:
    (a)   what you noticed
    (b)   how you initiated
    (c)   how you maintained the relationship.
    Is this a recognisable pattern?

■ Supplementary development of activity

1   Repeat steps 1 and 2 above but this time with the As finding another group's A, meeting up and relating to them. The Bs and Cs stay attached, as though appendages, to their group's A, supporting the shape initiated.
2   Repeat step 1 above but this time the two As find another two As from another group and relate to them. Bs and Cs stay supporting their own group's shape.
3   Repeat above until all As in the group are relating/interacting (non-verbally) with their supporters (Bs and Cs).

■ Additional outcomes

1 An awareness of feeling unique yet conforming to the group.
2 Acknowledgement of and support for the uniqueness of self.
3 An improvised choreography which the group maintains.

See p.168 for this activity used in another stage.

DEVELOPMENT OF THEME

SHAPES 3

Aims: To move within a group, initiating and maintaining a relationship with each other

Population: Adults
Conditions: None
Time: 8–10 minutes
Equipment: Music
Structure: Two groups

■ Activity

1 Divide into two groups and label selves A, B, C etc.
2 To the accompaniment of music, A goes into the centre of the group and makes a shape (see Section 2, 'Laban movement analysis'); then, by stretching, reaching and twisting, they move into a second shape.
3 As they make their transition from the first shape to the second, person B joins in and moves to make a linked shape with A's second shape.
4 Then A and B move together slowly to make a third shape, while person C joins in.
5 Keep moving and incorporate each group member until a mobile sculpture evolves, where all the group are moving and connecting, filling spaces and levels.
6 Bring it to a close at the end of the music by asking the group to find a final shape and freeze.

SHAPES 4

Aims: To introduce emotions and their associated postures
Population: All
Conditions: None
Time: 5 minutes
Equipment: None
Structure: Twos, threes

■ **Activity**

1 Ask each group to suggest an emotion to you. Label group members 1 and 2 (and 3 if in threes).
2 Explain that you will call out one of these emotions in turn and each no. 1 will respond with a reflection of the emotions in a posture.
3 Each no. 2 supports the posture with their own posture, followed by no. 3.
4 Change numbers in the group and repeat with next emotion.

TRUST 2

Aim: To develop trust
Population: All
Conditions: Safety ground rule
Time: 5–10 minutes
Equipment: None
Structure: Threes

■ Activity

1 Catch a middle person who decides when they will fall between the two others standing either side.
2 Ensure the catchers stand safely to receive the weight. One will catch the faller from behind, one from in front.
3 Change roles and each have turn as different catcher and as faller.
4 Extend space gradually between faller and catchers.

■ Supplementary development of activity

1 Repeat above, but with faller's eyes closed.
2 Repeat above, but with faller passive. Catchers catch and push back to other catcher rather than to middle balance position.

■ Additional outcomes

1 Excitement at risk taking.
2 Confidence at ability to support others.

TRUST 3

Aim: To develop ability to 'let go' of others and 'catch' self and others
Population: All
Conditions: Safety rule
Time: 15–25 minutes
Equipment: None
Structure: Threes

■ Activity

1   No. 1 (faller) faces no. 2 (holder) and takes wrist contact with opposite hand, holding no. 2 and leaning back so that weight is taken by contact. No. 3 (catcher) takes up position close behind no. 1.
2   Faller then counts '1, 2, 3' then lets go of wrist of no. 2 and is caught by no. 3.
3   Reverse roles so all take turn in each of the three roles.
4   In threes, discuss each role—how was it to be in each, for each person?

■ Supplementary development of activity

1   Repeat above, but with no. 2 counting '1, 2, 3' and letting go of faller. Holder takes opposite wrist of faller who does not hold on. Repeat with faller's eyes closed. Repeat without catcher (faller has to catch self).
2   Repeat 1–3, but with faller's eyes closed. Repeat without catcher.

■ Additional outcomes

1   Development of free flow to bound flow (see Section 2, 'Laban movement analysis').
2   Taking risks and containing self.

TRUST 4

Aim: To engender group trust
Population: All
Conditions: Safety rules, early in sessions
Time: 10–15 minutes
Equipment: None
Structure: Whole group

■ **Activity**

1 Group stand in circle, close together, shoulder to shoulder, hands flat and at shoulder height, one foot in front of other.
2 Volunteer (faller) stands rigid in centre and falls towards others who catch them gently and slowly by their shoulder blades and move them across to next person in circle.
3 Change volunteer.

■ **Supplementary development of activity**

1 Repeat, volunteer with eyes closed.
2 Repeat with more distance between catchers and fallers.
3 Could begin by requesting that volunteer decides when to fall and where. Catchers simply place them back in centre after each fall.
4 Repeat with fallers deciding to sink into floor, roll and get up, before falling against others again. Catchers support all movements.

■ **Additional outcomes**

1 Physical contact for whole group.
2 'Letting go' in the group.
3 Being moved by others.
4 Self-trust.

RHYTHM 7

Aim: To create a rhythmical movement phrase
Population: All
Conditions: None
Time: 5–10 minutes
Equipment: None
Structure: Whole group

■ Activity

1 Leader or group member suggests several words or phrases in turn.
2 Participants as a group chant and clap them out.
3 Participants select one of the words or phrases to individually move to in rhythm. Break it down into syllables.
4 In partners, share the moving rhythm—partner tries to guess which word/phrase it is based on.

LEVEL 4

Aims: To promote wider vocabulary of movement and adaptation of movements to different levels (see Glossary)
Population: Children
Conditions: None
Time: 2–3 minutes
Equipment: None
Structure: Individually

■ Activity

1 Leader suggests the upper part of the body is opened and stretched at a specific level (see Glossary); for example, stretching out arms horizontally while standing would be a stretch at the medium level.
2 Repeat this opening movement with the upper body, but at another level; for example, the same stretch as above while lying down.
3 Now close and curl the upper part of the body at a specified level.
4 Repeat this closing movement at another level.

■ Supplementary development of activity

1 Close upper and open lower part of the body, each at different levels, for example twist and hug the upper body while standing with feet wide apart.
2 Open upper and close lower part of the body, each at different levels.

■ Additional outcomes

Co-ordination between upper and lower parts of the body.

See p. 287 for this activity used in another stage.

LEVEL 5

Aim: To promote adaptability in movement
Population: All
Conditions: Mats underneath groups, safety element emphasised
Time: 5–10 minutes
Equipment: Mats
Structure: Groups of four to eight

■ Activity

1 Leader suggests group size, depending on age/functioning.
2 A volunteer lies down on back and the group carefully kneel each side, hands joining in criss-cross pattern, wrist to wrist under shoulders, hips and legs of volunteer.
3 Leader ensures firm support (including the head and arms) before group lift volunteer to a high level, above the supporters' heads if possible.
4 They keep the support and hold the volunteer at a low level before carefully placing them on the ground.

■ Supplementary development of activity

1 A swaying movement at both levels may be made by group if safe support is still possible.
2 Whole group help to lift and lower a volunteer.

■ Additional outcomes

1 Volunteer experiences their supported body at two levels.
2 Group experience their ability to work together to support the full body weight of the member.

LEVEL 6

Aim: To promote development of internal structure
Population: Children
Conditions: Warmed up physically
Time: 2–3 minutes
Equipment: Lively music
Structure: Individually

■ Activity

1 Leader suggests a practice activity, jumping, then jumping and turning in the air. Teach 'giving in to the floor' on landing from jumps.
2 Exploration of jumping and turning at high, medium and low levels follows.
3 Each participant makes a short 'jumping and turning' dance; i.e. they select three or four movements they like to make and put them together, flowing from one to the next.

■ Supplementary development of activity

1 Share the finished dance in threes.
2 Find a way for the three dances to be joined together so that they are integrated.

■ Additional outcomes

1 Creation of own structure for a particular movement activity at different levels.
2 Some energising of the group as a whole.

PRE-LATERALITY 2

Aim: Body awareness
Population: All
Conditions: None
Time: 5–6 minutes
Equipment: Ribbon, material
Structure: Individually, partners

■ **Activity**

1 Lying on back, move in co-ordination arms and legs, opening and closing; leader directs.
2 The partner who is lying watches the partner who is standing up in front of them and copies movement of arms and legs as though a mirror.
3 Leader may suggest shaking of one hand, kicking one leg as well as two arms and/or two legs moving together.
4 Partner is only to use one side of body now—identify by tying material, ribbon, or giving to hold.
5 Change roles.

■ **Supplementary development of activity**

1 Repeat 1–5 with both standing up facing each other.
2 Repeat 1–5 with one behind the other.
3 Repeat 1–5 with partners side by side.

■ **Additional outcomes**

Stress of one side of the body and then the other.

See p.190 for this activity used in another stage.

PRE-LATERALITY 3

Aim: To restrict movement to one side of the body, not crossing mid-line

Population: Children

Conditions: None

Time: 3 minutes

Equipment: Marker pens

Structure: Individually, partners

■ **Activity**

1 Leader tells group, 'imagine you had an opportunity to drive a car'.
2 The group then mime, with leader direction, getting into the car and starting it up.
3 Tell the group members that they are not allowed to turn the wheel so far round that their arms cross over their body mid-line; identify this by shirt buttons, etc.
4 Give them directions as though map reading to a blind driver, e.g. 'turn left slowly (big bend), straight on down the hill, turn sharp right, over traffic lights, stop, straight on, round the roundabout to the right, then come off to the left'.
5 Perhaps give mark on a hand to help them distinguish right from left.
6 The group travel physically during mime.

■ **Supplementary development of activity**

Repeat 1–6 with partner in passenger seat giving map reading directions.

■ **Additional outcomes**

Identification of right from left in body and in movement.

BODY CONTROL 6

Aim: To develop response to others' needs
Population: All
Conditions: Well into session
Time: 10–15 minutes
Equipment: None
Structure: Individual, partners

■ Activity

1 Individually group members balance on parts of the body, changing point of contact with floor after each balance; movement flows on.
2 Partners (A and B). Partner A finds ways of assisting partner B in balances they choose. Leader teaches support of partner for safety.
3 Partners counterbalance each other so that they can sit down, wrists in contact with each other.
4 Explore in groups of three counterbalance ideas.

■ Additional outcomes

Sensitivity to own body weight and its supportive aspects.

FLOOR PATTERN 4

Aims: To develop spatial orientation, decision making, turn-taking, trust
Population: Children
Conditions: None
Time: 4 minutes
Equipment: None
Structure: Whole group

■ Activity

1 Group take up individual shapes.
2 Two volunteers act as travellers, one leading, one following, and move over, around and under others in twisting pathways, staying close together.
3 Group leader suggests a variety of speeds and methods of travel.
4 The one leading can decide to give follower the lead by taking on any other group member's shape. That group member then becomes the follower.

■ Supplementary development of activity

1 Have three or four volunteers as the travellers.
2 Perhaps add music to accompany the dancing journey.

■ Additional outcomes

Tolerance of frustration for those not immediately chosen to become followers.

DEVELOPMENT OF THEME
(use in conjunction with 'floor pattern 3' in
introduction to theme)

FLOOR PATTERN 5

Aims: To arrive/leave with a flexible pathway
Population: All
Conditions: Beginning of group series/end of group series
Time: 10–15 minutes
Equipment: None
Structure: Individuals, partners

■ Activity

1 Each participant takes a circular, meandering pathway towards a space/object/person. Repeat for 3 minutes, travelling through several paths.
2 Select three pathways to approach and leave spaces/ objects/people. Travel in variety of ways across floor.
3 Rehearse each pathway and put them together to make a dance that focuses on arrival at and leaving the selected spaces/objects/people.
4 Share in twos the final pathway.
5 Discuss in twos what was noticed about partner's approach and arrival, then departure from selected places.

■ Supplementary development of activity

1 Whole group discussion about flexibility of approach and departure and what that conjures up for participants about their expectations for the group.
2 Explore direct pathways to/from places.

■ Additional outcomes

1 Arrival/departure issues acknowledged.
2 Contrasting pathways explored.

IMAGERY

Aims: To engage with an image through movement; to stimulate the imagination; to encourage spontaneous movement

Population: All
Conditions: None
Time: 15–20 minutes
Equipment: None
Structure: Individual, small groups

■ Activity

1 Leader draws an image and shows it to the group, who then respond to it in movement for 20 seconds or so.
2 Leader folds up pieces of paper with drawn/written images upon them; each member selects one, then for 2 minutes explores the image in movement.
3 Repeat step 2.
4 With a partner, try to guess the image from the movement responses.
5 Now each partner gives an image in turn for partner to respond to for 20 seconds. The image is given verbally, e.g. 'move like a lion sneaking up on a deer'.

■ Supplementary development of activity

1 In small groups, the leader secretly gives a visual or verbal image to each group.
2 Each group spends 4 minutes preparing to respond.
3 Each group shares their response with the whole group who may guess the image given.

■ Additional outcomes

Development of symbolic expression, use of expressive movement in communication, development of a specific theme which the group is addressing, introduction of a relevant theme for the group.

See p.174 for this activity used in another stage.

DEVELOPMENT OF THEME

BALANCE 5

Aim: To reduce impulsivity
Population: All
Conditions: Adolescents may find blindfold more difficult
Time: 4–5 minutes
Equipment: Music, blindfold
Structure: Individually

■ **Activity**

1 As in the game of 'statues', move with the music and freeze in a balance when it stops.
2 Leader identifies balance at first, e.g. with one leg stretched behind.
3 Ask for a volunteer to 'stop' the music (with their back to the group).
4 Change volunteers.
5 After several turns, each member to create own balance.
6 On the 'stop', each member holds balance for 5 seconds, looks around and selects a balance from group for their next choice of balance.

■ **Supplementary development of activity**

Repeat 1–4 blindfolded.

■ **Additional outcomes**

1 Grounds group and focuses them on centring themselves (see Glossary).
2 Awareness of own and others' creativity.
3 Control of self and others (especially music operator).

See p.147 for this activity used in another stage.

DEVELOPMENT OF THEME

TENSION-RELAXATION 1

Aim: To use imagination in association with tension-release activity
Population: Children, adolescents
Conditions: None
Time: 3 minutes
Equipment: None
Structure: Individual

■ Activity

1 Move like 'Action Man' with strong, jerky actions.
2 Transform into 'floppy doll' with flaccid movements.
3 Have group go from one interpretation to the other rapidly in turn (e.g. 10 seconds in each alternately).

■ Additional outcomes

Adaptation in movement.

TENSION-RELAXATION 2

Aims: To promote body sensation and self-trust
Population: All
Conditions: Warmed up
Time: 3–4 minutes
Equipment: None
Structure: Individual

■ Activity

1 Sitting with one leg bent under hips, gently support self as you lie back slowly.
2 Feel muscles in thigh stretching, breathe out as though into them and relax back on elbows.
3 If able, go further back for 30 seconds and watch breath.
4 Slowly come back up to sitting and repeat on other side.

DEVELOPMENT OF THEME

QUALITY 7

Aim: To develop quality of strength
Population: All
Conditions: None
Time: 2–5 minutes
Equipment: None
Structure: Individual, group

■ Activity

1 Leader suggests a mime of pushing a car out of the mud.
2 Group form themselves together in preparation for mime, expressing strength in legs and lower body and shoulders and arms.
3 Group carry out the mime (in roles of either 'pushers' or 'car').
4 Group can release the strength at the point they choose, or imagine an ending (e.g. the car not shifting; a sudden shift as it moves off; or a slow release as it is pushed on through and out of mud).

QUALITY 8

Aim: To develop quality of lightness
Population: All
Conditions: None
Time: 10 minutes
Equipment: Pieces of light material
Structure: Individual

■ **Activity**

1 Leader distributes pieces of material.
2 Suggest group walk quietly without disturbing the material held by two corners in front/to side of body.
3 Moving in different directions with other movements, trying to retain material as still.
4 Throw the material and echo with body the way it falls to the floor.

QUALITY 9

Aim: To develop quality of lightness
Population: All
Conditions: None
Time: 2–3 minutes
Equipment: None
Structure: Individual, pairs

■ **Activity**

1 Leader suggests group move as though the air under their arms is sustaining them, as though gravity did not exist, like moon-walking.

2 In pairs, mime pumping the air into balloons under partner's arms. They then move as though lifted up and floating away. Partner then decides what happens next; for example, as though air was seeping out? as though the balloon had burst? Tell your partner what is to happen and they move in response.

DEVELOPMENT OF THEME

QUALITY 10

Aim: To develop quality of suddenness
Population: All
Conditions: None
Time: 3 minutes
Equipment: Wooden block or drum
Structure: Individual

■ Activity

Group move hands and feet sharply in time to a tapping rhythm given by leader on block or drum.

QUALITY 11

Aim: To develop quality of lightness
Population: All
Conditions: None
Time: 2 minutes
Equipment: None
Structure: Whole group

■ Activity

1 Group make circle, walk into centre as though on egg-shells. Try not to break the shells.
2 Move out to edge of circle again and repeat, focusing on careful, light steps, air under arms, chest light.

QUALITY 12

Aim: To develop quality of sustained movement
Population: All
Conditions: None
Time: 2 minutes
Equipment: None
Structure: Individual

■ Activity

1 Imagine a waterfall; the movement is continuous.
2 Move as though you are the water, in continual motion, whether as a trickle or rushing over boulders and cliffs.
3 Now move at half the speed.
4 Now, as though in slow-motion film, half as slow again.

■ Additional outcomes

Develops continuity of movement.

QUALITY 13

Aim: To develop quality of sustained movement
Population: All
Conditions: None
Time: 3 minutes
Equipment: None
Structure: Pairs

■ Activity

1 Leader suggests each pair select a game together (e.g. tennis).
2 Mime the game in slow motion.
3 Share with another pair, who have to guess the game.

WHISPERS

Aim: To practice imitation skills
Population: Adolescents, adults
Conditions: None
Time: 5 minutes
Equipment: None
Structure: Whole group or several small groups

■ **Activity**

1. Group in circle standing one behind the other.
2. Leader gives instructions that each person should imitate any movement, however slight, that they notice the person in front making. No one, however, is to move purposefully, other than to imitate the person in front.
3. The leader makes one purposeful movement to begin the group movement. The person behind the leader repeats it so that the movement is passed around the circle.
4. Allow group to experience the movements that evolve from all the unconscious movement emitted from members.

■ **Additional outcomes**

Awareness of how much movement we generate without full consciousness.

See p.170 for this activity used in another stage.

DIRECTIONALITY 2

Aim: To create a self-initiated structure
Population: All
Conditions: None
Time: 4 minutes
Equipment: Music of their choice
Structure: Individual

■ **Activity**

1 Leader suggests that participants find a space for themselves.
2 While in that space, travel forwards, backwards, sideways and turn in various combinations.
3 Select several directions and create a repeatable but simple sequence of movement with the music as an accompaniment.

PLANES 1

Aims: To explore preferences and develop non-habitual movement pattern

Population: All
Conditions: None
Time: 5 minutes
Equipment: None
Structure: Individual, partners

■ Activity

1 Rise and sink to and from the high level (see Glossary).
2 Open and close at the medium level.
3 Forward and backward rolls at the low level.
4 Explore the plane(s) that are the most difficult or unusual for you to move within.
5 Begin with movement in one of the 'easiest' planes and add on movement from step 4 above to make a growth sequence.
6 Think of a word to describe the transition from the 'easy' to the more difficult/unusual planes.
7 Share movement and word with a partner.

■ Supplementary development of activity

Discussion of habits and patterns in movement preferences, reference to the transition phase when attempting change.

PLANES 2

Aim: To provide clear phrasing from a rhythmical structure
Population: Children
Conditions: Warmed up, especially in feet and legs
Time: 3–4 minutes
Equipment: None
Structure: Individual

■ Activity

1 Leader suggests a movement phrase such as 'jump, jump, jump, jump; turn, turn, turn; jump and turn, jump and turn, jump and turn'.
2 Leader then suggests participants make up own rhythms, using jump and turn.

■ Additional outcomes

Energises group.

TENSION-RELAXATION 3

Aims: To release tension, co-operation, change of tension
Population: Not groups that are known to be violent
Conditions: Safety rules reiterated
Time: 3–4 minutes
Equipment: Possibly percussion
Structure: Small groups

■ **Activity**

1 In small groups, interpret a volcano exploding.
2 Build up tension slowly, using vocalisation if appropriate.
3 Explode outwards, move through imaginary stages of lava slowly flowing then solidifying like a rock formation (stillness).
4 Share each group's interpretation.
5 Do as a whole group.

PASS

Aim: To become aware of sound and movement in group
Population: All
Conditions: None
Time: 10 minutes
Equipment: Music
Structure: Group

■ **Activity**

1 Pass a sound around circle.
2 Pass a movement around circle.
3 With music to accompany the group, they follow leader's movement until the leader says 'pass'; then next one on right develops that movement for a while. When they feel group is following it okay, they then say 'pass', and so on.

DEVELOPMENT OF THEME

CLAP

Aims: To let go of control in group and allow the group to develop own structures
Population: All
Conditions: None
Time: 10 minutes
Equipment: None
Structure: Whole group

■ Activity

1 Begin by telling group they will make a group rhythm through clapping, sound-making and movement—a group improvisation (6 minutes).
2 Leader asks for people to indicate if they believe they are not rhythmical, suggests that this activity may show that they are.
3 Begin with each member making their own clapping sound at random, simultaneously, in the circle. Closing eyes sometimes helps overcome inhibitions.
4 Let the clapping stimulate 'stamping' movement across the centre of the circle, voice sounds etc. Leader may have to 'hold' the experience, participating and picking up on rhythms as they emerge.
5 Allow ending to be spontaneous.

DEVELOPMENT OF THEME

PERCUSSION

Aims: Impulse control, taking initiatives
Population: Children, adolescents
Conditions: None
Time: 15–25 minutes
Equipment: Variety of percussion instruments
Structure: Individual and two groups

■ Activity

1 Participants asked to explore the sound their selected instrument makes. Leader to guide this.
2 As a group, can only move when an individual initiates a sound. Freeze if someone else then comes in with their sound.
3 Leader can say 'change' and/or call out names to play sounds for a while, then encourage individuals to take own initiative.

■ Supplementary development of activity

1 Suggest one group become the orchestra and the other the movers. The sound then accompanies the movement (which could be rehearsed first for 5 minutes). Give 3 minutes for this. Change over roles.
2 Suggest they now use sound as the stimulus for the movement. Orchestra plays and the movers dance out the music. (NB Movers need to be encouraged to interact as a group in the dance.)

■ Additional outcomes

1 A self-initiated group choreography with own musical accompaniment.
2 Self-confidence in movement.

COLOURS 1

Aims: To work with colour in movement and explore our feelings in relation to colour

Population: All
Conditions: None
Time: 20–30 minutes
Equipment: None
Structure: Individual and group

■ **Activity**

1 Leader suggests group move for 10 seconds to each of the following colours; red, green, blue, yellow, pink etc.
2 Ask group to call out own choices.
3 In pairs; one moves to a colour of their choice, the other guesses it.
4 Three groups; leader gives a colour to each group who then have 1 minute to rehearse its expression as a group, then perform it. Other groups guess the colour.
5 Each group thinks of own colour, rehearses and performs it for others to guess.

COLOURS 2

Aims: To work with colour in movement and explore our feelings in relation to colour

Population: All

Conditions: None

Time: 20–30 minutes

Equipment: Paper and felt-tip pens

Structure: Individual

■ Activity

1 Close eyes; imagine colour yellow; you are moving in yellowness.
2 This gradually changes from a dark yellow to misty to white (give a couple of minutes in each shade).
3 Gradually visualise out of the white a colour that is soothing for you.
4 Bring it out, dance with it, play and enjoy it (3 minutes).
5 Say goodbye to the colour, knowing it is always there for you.
6 Draw your colour dance.
7 Share picture in large group feedback.

COLOURS 3

Aims: To work with colour in movement and explore our feelings in relation to colour
Population: All
Conditions: None
Time: 1 hour
Equipment: Paper and felt-tip pens
Structure: Individual and groups

■ Activity

1   Select either red, yellow or green and make a picture of one of these colours (using all colours you like) to depict emotions and associations.
2   Walk round all pictures and write on slips of paper your associations and your guess of which colour it depicts. Put paper under picture.
3   Return to your own picture and put colour and association on piece of paper at top of picture.
4   Walk round all pictures again reading these.
5   Walk to next picture along from yours. Make a movement that expresses all of it or some aspect of it. Move to the next with that movement and do the same. If you meet anyone, interact with them as you go. Make it flow. This is a group dance of all your perceptions of these colours.
6   Return to your own picture, read the words underneath. Share in pairs what you have found and any connections between what your colour was expressing and others' perceptions.
7   Group sharing of dance pictures and thoughts.

■ Supplementary development of activity

1   All 'reds', 'yellows' and 'greens' could meet and, using their pictures as guides, dance out the colour.
2   Share dance with other groups.

DARKNESS AND LIGHT

Aim: To become aware of blind spots
Population: Adults
Conditions: Well-established group
Time: 20 minutes
Equipment: Paper and felt-tip pens
Structure: Individual

■ Activity

1 Draw an image that is to do with darkness and light (4 minutes).
2 Using the picture as a map, move from the darkness to the light (4 minutes).
3 In fours or fives; select one aspect of the improvisation you would like to explore further with the group's support. Group will give help in movement and sound to enable that individual really to dance out that aspect.
4 Discuss in turn your feelings, memories, images and any other connections you may have made for yourself.

■ Supplementary development of activity

Individual could repeat the dance with any new awareness.

WE ARE OUR BODIES 1

Aim: To sense our body image
Population: All
Conditions: When group is well established
Time: 1 hour
Equipment: Large roll of paper, felt-tip pens, paint, crayons
Structure: Individual, pairs, whole group

■ **Activity**

1 In a group mingle together, meet each other in turn (leader says 'change') and say one thing about your body to partner, starting with the words 'I am ...'
2 Now repeat, but express one thing you notice about your partner's body.
3 Collect paper and cut it to the length you believe your body to be (do not measure it up against you first).
4 Meditation preparation (5 minutes); have them sit near their paper in a comfortable position, eyes closed if possible. Draw their attention to breath, floor, body in contact with itself and floor. Move on to talk about the 'sense of body self'. Ask them to reflect upon how they care for their bodies, clothe them, take part in physical activities; what about sexuality? Breathe deeply five times and open eyes.
5 Suggest they draw a portrait of their bodies on the paper (15 minutes).
6 Put the portrait up on the wall.
7 Stand back 1.5 or 1.8 metres and look at it. For 15 minutes, allow and receive the dance within you as it begins to move in response to the portrait. Follow the impulses to move.
8 Re-make the essence of that dance for 2 minutes. Draw it on a small sheet of paper, give it a title.
9 Turn portrait around towards wall.

10 In pairs, in turn, share essence of dance. Partner draws what he observes during/after dance. Give it a title. 2 minutes each, no talking.

11 Discuss in same pairs the similarities/differences in the drawings.

DEVELOPMENT OF THEME

WE ARE OUR BODIES 2

Aim: To sense our body image
Population: All
Conditions: When group is well established
Time: 1 hour
Equipment: Large roll of paper, felt-tip pens, paint, crayons
Structure: Individual, pairs, whole group

■ Activity

1 Take portrait and use marks to illustrate where non-functional areas are, e.g. weakness, strengths, hot, cold, associations.
2 Mark your portrait with a colour, shape and quality that is expressive of these.
3 Select one mark and make a movement to symbolise it.
4 Allow the movement to become a sensation in that area of your body. Close eyes and take a few minutes to sense this area. Breathe slowly and deeply.
5 Let torso begin to move slightly to express the sensation.
6 Repeat several times, noticing the quality and shape of movement. Does the movement want to take you across the space? What is the rhythm? Are there any images appearing, sounds, words?
7 Remember the mark; does the movement still fit? Let it develop so you are able to express it clearly. Exaggerate its shape.
8 In fours, share main aspect of your 'mark dance'. Others give feedback in non-critical manner.
9 Performer takes 2 minutes to draw anything that comes to mind afterwards. Meanwhile next one is sharing their dance.
10 All complete sentence, 'my body is telling me ...'
11 Share in large group the pictures and sentences.

12 Closure (individually): close eyes, suggest they breathe slowly noticing the breath coming in through the nose and out through the mouth, and talk them through a grounding of body, i.e. in contact with the floor, how far from walls, door, back to the self.

■ Supplementary development of activity

See *We are our bodies 1.* Use that activity as a supplementary development to the above.

HAND DANCES

Aim: To become aware of self with another in movement
Population: All
Conditions: None
Time: 10 minutes
Equipment: Music (classical guitar)
Structure: Pairs

■ Activity

1 In pairs, sit opposite each other, close eyes and make contact with left wrists.
2 Explore space between you while maintaining a protective space for yourself.
3 After 3–4 minutes have the pairs stand up while maintaining the contact.
4 Now have them change wrists without losing contact.
5 Now have them travel forward/backwards/sideways. Who initiates? How does this affect your space?
6 After 10 minutes have them find a way to come to a resolution.

■ Additional outcomes

Awareness of personal space needs.

STILLNESS IN MOVEMENT

Aim: To enable group to become aware of group's theme(s) in movement

Population: Adolescents, adults

Conditions: None

Time: 5–10 minutes

Equipment: None

Structure: Whole group (minimum 3)

■ Activity

1 Stand in a circle, one behind the other.
2 Simply watch the person in front of you and move in precisely the same way that they do (NB No one is to move consciously—shadow movements only).

■ Additional outcomes

1 Extension of normal movement range.
2 Awareness of group tension.

INTERPERSONAL

Aim: To become aware of self in relation to others
Population: Adults
Conditions: Long attention span required
Time: 45 minutes
Equipment: None
Structure: Individual

■ Activity

1 Move with the sensation you feel in your body, e.g. lightness, agility, resistance, heaviness. You are as if alone, encountering yourself moving.
2 Use familiar movements to make a pathway around the space.
3 Repeat patterning and movements so that you know them. There is a beginning, a middle and an end. Do not acknowledge or communicate with any people or objects. Maintain an inward frame of mind.
4 What are the bodily sensations you notice while on this journey? Enlarge these sensations and express them in movement.
5 Now repeat pathway three times and exaggerate your movements. Return to beginning of pathway, close eyes in that space and remember the path.
6 Now repeat pathway three times but notice other people/ objects as you go. Who do you notice on your pathway? Continue your journey, being aware of any bodily sensations and movement, and if they change as you notice others. Who do you select to notice? Do not interact, just notice. Exaggerate those changes in body sensation as expressed in movement. Return to the beginning of your pathway, close eyes and replay the journey.
7 Now repeat the pathway three times, this time interacting with others. Who do you choose and who chooses you? Do you initiate or do they? Who leaves first?

Notice your body sensations and movement. Exaggerate any changes you are aware of. Return to beginning of pathway and close eyes, remembering journey.

8 Again travel pathway three times but only noticing others. What/who do you notice? What is the body/movement like now; any differences? Exaggerate them. Return and remember.

9 Alone again, travel your pathway for the last time (three times) and notice how the frame of mind manifests itself in your movement. Is it different from the last time you were alone on your pathway? Return and remember.

10 Take a sheet of paper with five columns, headed:
(a) 'when I am alone',
(b) 'when I notice',
(c) 'when I interact',
(d) 'when I notice again',
(e) 'when I'm alone again'.
Brainstorm for 1 minute per column anything you remember: words, sensations, movements, experience, actions, feelings, thoughts, images.

11 In pairs, discuss experiences from each column and relate to life events.

■ Supplementary development of activity

1 Before any discussion in pairs, you could select one word from each column and share it in hand gesture. Do not let your partner see the words. Make hands express sensation, etc.

2 Partner (a) guesses the word; (b) replies in hand gesture using their selection of words from same columns.

3 Interact together in hand dance, using any of the selected words as starting-points. Keep to movement repertoire already experienced.

4 Complete the following sentence individually: 'My body tells me ...'

5 Select one of the columns and draw a picture that expresses it.

6 Large group discussion and sharing of picture.

SHAPING SPACE

Aim: To explore the relationship you have with space, and it with you

Population: Any experienced movement group

Conditions: None

Time: 10–15 minutes

Equipment: None

Structure: Individual

■ Activity

1 Move as though in a space that is
   (a) tight,
   (b) narrow,
   (c) convex,
   (d) concave,
   (e) overhanging,
   (f) steep,
   (g) towering,
   (h) very expansive (e.g. a plain).
2 Using the expansive space as a starting-point, guide movers from the grassy plain into the air, up and away from the land to the heavens and outer space.
3 Guide them into a 'planet dance', which takes place in Father Sky but returns to Mother Earth in a group, and let them sway together.
4 Finish with a grounding (see Glossary) or centring (see Glossary) of the group. For example, sitting cross-legged, being aware of spine, seat bones and breath.
5 Discuss the 'planet dance' as a group.

■ Supplementary development of activity

1 Select one aspect of your experience of moving in space and make a picture of it (5 minutes). Give the picture a title.

2 In threes; one moves to express their picture and others share what it felt like to watch them (no critical comments).

LINES 2

Aim: To interact with partner
Population: All
Conditions: Early sessions
Time: 10 minutes
Equipment: Paper and felt-tip pens
Structure: Pairs

■ Activity

1 Make markings on the paper together and explore qualities of line.
2 Now, with a clean sheet of paper, use marking of lines to interact in a line conversation.
3 Use the drawing as a map for having a movement conversation together.

■ Supplementary development of activity

5 minutes to reflect upon the experience and state what was appreciated and resented about the last interaction.

■ Additional outcomes

Awareness of what we say to each other using non-verbal media only.

RELATIONSHIP 5

Aims: To observe and respond to another in movement
Population: Adolescents, adults
Conditions: Some improvisation skills
Time: 3–5 minutes
Equipment: Music of choice
Structure: Pairs

■ **Activity**

1 With a partner, mirror or contrast movements and have a movement conversation or argument (30 seconds).
2 What were the words or phrases that could describe the experience (discuss for 1 minute)?
3 Repeat conversation, allowing words to accompany movement.
4 In what ways do you normally enhance your communication (words and movement)? Ask for feedback from partner.

■ **Additional outcomes**

1 Insights into mismatching of words and movement in communication.
2 How misunderstandings can arise in the 'reading' of body movement.
3 Awareness of authentic movement supporting words.

RELATIONSHIP 6

Aim: To develop leadership qualities
Population: All
Conditions: None
Time: 2–3 minutes
Equipment: None
Structure: One or two groups and volunteer

■ Activity

1 One member volunteers to conduct the group, using hands, giving non-verbal signals to promote a movement activity (for example, arms up and down quickly to promote jumping).
2 Discuss the group's interpretation of the signals.

■ Supplementary development of activity

Conduct two groups simultaneously, using left and right hands to give signals.

RELATIONSHIP 7

Aims: To encourage meeting and parting
Population: Children, adolescents
Conditions: When maintaining relationships is difficult.
Ensure safety rules (not to let go of elastic)
Time: 2–3 minutes
Equipment: Elastic, 2.5–5 centimetres wide, 1.5–1.8 metres
long, hand hole securely sewn in each end.
Plenty of space
Structure: Pairs

■ Activity

1 Using the elastic to link partners, suggest moving apart and running together so they pass each other.
2 Vary side of body passed (e.g. right sides and left sides).
3 As they run towards each other, elastic shrinks, then stretches as they part again, allowing for tension that encourages a recoil again for a return to the meeting place.

■ Supplementary development of activity

Perhaps make noise as they run.

■ Additional outcomes

1 Tension-relaxation.
2 Separation, yet linked in relationship.
3 Co-operation.

RELATIONSHIP 8

Aim: To relate to objects
Population: All
Conditions: Confidence in improvisation
Time: 2 minutes
Equipment: Any appropriate prop
Structure: Individual

■ Activity

1 Approach and make contact with the prop.
2 Explore it in movement.
3 Move with it for 40 seconds.
4 Leave the prop.

■ Supplementary development of activity

1 Discuss the qualities of the prop in pairs.
2 Share your 40 seconds dance with your partner.

RELATIONSHIP 9

Aim: To express anger
Population: Adolescents
Conditions: Safety rules reiterated, small group
Time: 1–2 minutes
Equipment: Soft beach balls, large wall space (no windows)
Structure: Individual

■ Activity

1 Each member faces the wall area (well defined) and throws the ball hard against it.
2 Repeat for 1 minute, encourage use of sound as they throw.
3 Suggest they use words such as 'I hate ...'
4 Discuss in group.

RELATIONSHIP 10

Aims: Structuring and channelling energy
Population: All
Conditions: Safety structures
Time: Variable
Equipment: Mats/cushions
Structure: Whole group

■ Activity

1. Slap or bang hands on a mat/cushion with clear phrasing (e.g. bang, bang, BANG and stop).
2. Leader to maintain leadership role in channelling energy towards a resolution.

RELATIONSHIP 11

Aims: To identify and communicate needs
Population: All
Conditions: Able to work in small group without leader
Time: 5–10 minutes
Equipment: None
Structure: Small groups of three or four

■ Activity

1 Each member in turn asks group to do something for them, e.g. give them a swing, jump them high, a rock, a trust fall, etc.
2 Leader may have previously given opportunities for various small group activities; individuals select one they would especially like for themselves.
3 Leader must be conscious of over-ambitious groups, for example, with regard to carrying, catching and ensuring safety aspects are adhered to (how to carry, hold safely another human being).

■ Supplementary development of activity

1 Perhaps then engage whole group in doing something for someone.
2 Leader could ask group to give them a rock or ride of some sort.

RELATIONSHIP 12

Aim: Nurturing a partner
Population: All
Conditions: None
Time: 5–6 minutes
Equipment: Mats
Structure: Threes

■ Activity

1 Two kneel down opposite each other; the third lies between them and is rolled carefully from one set of knees across to the other.
2 Change roles so all have a turn in the middle.

RELATIONSHIP 13

Aims: Trust and letting go
Population: All
Conditions: None
Time: Variable
Equipment: None
Structure: Threes

■ Activity

1 . In threes, standing, two catchers face each other with the third, who is to be pivoted and rocked back and forth between them, in the middle.
2 Distance between the two catchers depends on the group's needs, but begin fairly close so there is not too far for the middle one to fall.
3 Middle one remains rigid, like a metal rod, and is passive. Catchers use wide stance, knees bent and hands wide open to receive weight. Contact shoulder blades and upper chest.
4 Change roles.

■ Supplementary development of activity

Middle one decides when to rock back and forth, taking an active role.

DIRECTIONALITY 3

Aim: To experience the backward direction (into the unknown)

Population: All (must have some ego)

Conditions: Emphasis on safety ground rules

Time: 10–35 minutes

Equipment: None

Structure: Individually and partners

■ Activity

1 Individually walk backwards from one side of space to other. Slowly move with eyes fixed on object in front, be aware of distance increasing as journey continues into the unknown—the future—backwards into the future.

2 In pairs; roles of 'wise guide' (super ego) and 'journeyer'. Wise guide supports partner as they move backwards by standing in front and using voice and/or touch to help them on their journey.

3 Next have participants put out chairs and other objects in the space. Repeat journey, the partner acting as guide.

4 Repeat journey with guide behind journeyer (if contact is made with others by journeyer, help journeyer to explore these others gently).

5 Change roles.

■ Supplementary development of activity

1 Repeat 1–5 above, but journeyer closes eyes.

2 Could also repeat 2–5 but without 'wise guide'. Each participant is a combination of wise guide and journeyer.

■ Additional outcomes

1 Development of giving and receiving support/guidance from others.
2 Brings out the theme of the unknown, fear in exploration.
3 Encourages change of pace for under-bounded (see Glossary) groups.
4 Promotes sense of a base, and moving out from there to explore environment.
5 Can act as an integrator of the actor and observer roles.

BODY BOUNDARY 3

Aims: To give and receive peer attention, to develop trust, sensitivity and awareness of self affecting others

Population: Adolescents, adults

Conditions: Safety rules

Time: 10 minutes

Equipment: None

Structure: Partners in whole group

■ Activity

1 All stand in a circle.
2 Pummel all soft areas of own body and chest (making sound).
3 Turn to person (partner) on left and pummel with loose fists the other's calves, thighs, buttocks, backs, shoulders, upper arms.
4 Finish by stroking from the top of their head down to their feet slowly in one gentle sweep.
5 Turn to your right and repeat with that person.
6 Notice the differences in contact between the two people massaging you.
7 Notice your responses to them and any differences.

■ Supplementary development of activity

1 After the above, open up a large group discussion that encourages each person to give feedback to those who massaged them.
2 Ask how it felt to be getting and giving this kind of attention from each other.

■ Additional outcomes

A recognition of the part physical contact plays in their lives. A new level of relationship with peers. The ability to give and receive feedback from peers. Giving and receiving attention in a group.

See p.177 for this activity used in another stage.

BODY BOUNDARY 6

Aim: To let go enough to experience self and others
Population: Adults
Conditions: Middle to end of sessions
Time: 5 minutes
Equipment: None
Structure: Individual, pairs

■ Activity

1 Give yourself a hug while sitting down.
2 Repeat standing.
3 Give another group member a hug in the same manner as you gave yourself one.
4 Tell them how you experienced their hug.
5 Any ideas about how you took care of yourself?

■ Supplementary development of activity

Hug each member of the group in turn.

■ Additional outcomes

1 An increased sense of self.
2 Through this physical contact some issues may arise concerning their experience of being held or touched when an infant/child.
3 There may be an opening up to self-care and to caring for others.

See p. 303 for this activity used in another stage.

BODY BOUNDARY 7

Aims: To experience being moved and receiving that experience from others; to be in a moving relationship without any direct physical contact; to establish sense of self as separate from the environment

Population: All, particularly young children

Conditions: Before introducing touch

Time: 10 minutes

Equipment: Large pieces of strong material

Structure: Pairs, small groups

■ Activity

1 In pairs, one partner (volunteer) is wrapped in the material.
2 Partner spins, pulls and swings them, slowly at first.
3 Reverse roles of activator and volunteer and repeat.
4 Form small groups; give a volunteer a ride across the floor in the material.

■ Supplementary development of activity

1 Find a beginning, middle and end for the group process. Share your story with the whole group.
2 First volunteers, then activators, give comments to whole group.

Additional outcomes

1 Sense of being in receipt of a moving experience generated by peer(s).
2 Sense of body, since in contact with the floor through the material.
3 Free-flowing exercise.

BODY BOUNDARY 8

Aim: To encourage sense of self and others through whole bodily contact

Population: Adults, children

Conditions: After some physical contact has been introduced

Time: 15 minutes

Equipment: None

Structure: Pairs, whole group

■ Activity

1 Partners grip wrist to wrist as one slides partner across floor on their back. Give time for trust to build.
2 Ensure they feel their waist (centre) by wriggling the sliding partner.
3 Reverse roles.
4 Now both take up a long stretched rolling movement together, with hand to hand contact.
5 Practice rolling from one end of the space to the other in pairs.
6 Whole group positioned side by side prone on floor, partners head to head.
7 In turn, each pair roll over the whole group, trying to keep hands linked and rolling at the same time. Ensure no spaces between people on floor.

■ Supplementary development of activity

1 Slide partners towards a people pile in the centre of the space.
2 Roll together into a people pile. Ensure people are in contact with each other both during the making of the pile and at the finish.
3 Take a couple of minutes to relax as a whole group on each other's bodies.

4 Slowly roll away from each other into a space on your own. Notice the contact with the floor as opposed to people.

■ Additional outcomes

1 Development of group cohesion.
2 Sense of self as separate from others.
3 Active-passive experience.

BALANCE 7

Aims: Inner control, accepting a structure
Population: Children
Conditions: None
Time: 5 minutes
Equipment: None
Structure: Individual, pairs, small groups

■ Activity

1 Leader gives a balance position, which is held by all participants; e.g. two hands and one foot, seat, shoulders.
2 After, say, 5 seconds another balance is given.
3 Gradually make the balances more difficult, e.g. decrease the surface area in contact with the floor.
4 Repeat with a partner who is teaming up to make the given balance. Encourage physical contact.
5 Change partners on each balance.
6 Repeat in small groups.

■ Supplementary development of activity

1 Repeat whole exercise within a confined space, e.g. on a mat.
2 Travel in the balance to other end of room.

■ Additional outcomes

1 Can restrict impulsive action and act as a containment for hyperactivity.
2 Working with others to a given structure, problem solving.

DEVELOPMENT OF THEME

PERSONAL SPACE 6

Aim: Awareness of object world in relation to self
Population: All
Conditions: None
Time: 5 minutes
Equipment: Ball, mat, chair, bean bag, hoop
Structure: Individual

■ Activity

1 Place an object near to participant. Suggest they focus on object.
2 Suggest they move towards the object; ensure they are close but not touching the object.
3 Suggest they explore moving around it at first.
4 Develop the exploration by suggesting movement over, to one side, other side, in front of and behind the object at various distances but where they could still reach the object if need be.

■ Supplementary development of activity

1 Reach for, touch and grasp the object, integrating it into closer proximity of body exploring relationships in space with the object.
2 Grasp and let go of the object in personal space while remaining glued to one spot.
3 In twos, explore the object in own personal space; how it can be moved, related to, etc. Stay rooted to one place on floor. When the object is released by design or accident out of the place, the partner retrieves and continues exploration for themselves in the same manner in own personal space.
4 Leader could stipulate 30 seconds or 1 minute per person before change-over; could accompany with light piano music.

■ Additional outcomes

An awareness of objects in relation to manipulation skills within own space. Development of exploratory senses towards:

(a) moving an object in relation to the body and spaces created by the body

(b) moving the body in relation to a still object.

PERSONAL SPACE 7
(SLOW MOTION BOXING)

Aims: To move in and out of personal space
Population: Adolescents, particularly boys
Conditions: None
Time: 5 minutes
Equipment: Mats and sustained musical accompaniment
Structure: Pairs

■ Activity

1 Each pair on a mat, or in designated space, kneeling down facing each other. Leader suggests that a movement dialogue will take place between them for 30 seconds where no touching is allowed. The game is called 'slow motion boxing' and the idea is that one initiates a movement towards the other who responds by pulling away, then miming a movement back.
2 Falling sideways, backwards as a response can be encouraged.
3 Only allow, for example, four punches each to ensure that the slow motion element is adhered to.
4 They must contain the movement dialogue to the confined space (e.g. the mat).

■ Supplementary development of activity

1 Repeat half-kneeling.
2 Repeat standing.
3 Discussion could centre on control of fighting impulses, play fighting.
4 Teach 'how to fall' onto the floor.

■ Additional outcomes

Some awareness of body control, how to fall, and the relationship of mind to body in aggression.

BODY INVENTORY

Aims: To promote bodily and social awareness
Population: Children, adults
Conditions: Once trust and group cohesion are established
Time: 10 minutes
Equipment: None
Structure: Individual, partner, group

■ Activity

Leader calls out two body parts, e.g. ear to knee. Either part is moved towards the other part until they are in contact.

■ Supplementary development of activity

1   Have the individual travel with parts in contact.
2   Have people contact another person, part to part.
3   Have the whole group in physical contact and perform a task such as sitting, swaying, jumping without losing contact.
4   Could use same parts, e.g. feet to feet.

■ Additional outcomes

The group should begin to focus on and identify different body parts. The physical contact with others can enable a different sort of closeness in the group to emerge. Often laughter results from, say, travelling with parts in contact.

RELAXATION

Aim: To be aware of own body
Population: All except children
Conditions: None
Time: 10 minutes
Equipment: None
Structure: Individual

■ Activity

1 In a quiet room with softened lighting, lie on back, become aware of breathing.
2 Take in a few deep breaths and, while exhaling, mentally say the word 'relax'.
3 Concentrate on face and feel any tension in eyes and face. Let it relax and become comfortable, like a tight rubber band going limp. Feel this wave of relaxation through whole body.
4 Tense the eyes and face, grit teeth and then relax and feel it spread through body as a whole.
5 Repeat step 4 for each body part, moving from neck down to toes. Picture in mind tension and it melting away.
6 Rest for 2–5 minutes afterwards.
7 Let muscles and eyelids lighten up and become ready to open eyes, become aware of room.
8 Let eyes open and be ready to stand up.

PUSHING

Aims: To channel aggression, get a sense of own power
Population: All
Conditions: No violence
Time: 5 minutes
Equipment: None
Structure: Pairs

■ Activity

1   In pairs, push against each other, back to back, while sitting. Leader to count '5, 4, 3, 2, 1' for time allowed. Aim to push partner across floor.
2   Change partners.
3   Change to pushing hips to hips, shoulders to shoulders and hands to hands, in that order, each with a different partner.

■ Supplementary development of activity

1   One partner says 'yes' and one 'no' during the activity (pairs decide who says which).
2   Reflection upon what the conflict was like, which role you chose to play, etc.

■ Additional outcomes

1   Assertion.
2   Development of quality of strength and bound flow (see Section 2, 'Laban movement analysis').

DEVELOPMENT OF THEME

CO-OPERATION

Aim: To work together when touch is not appropriate
Population: All
Conditions: Safety
Time: 5 minutes
Equipment: Light garden sticks or canes; music if preferred
Structure: Pairs

■ **Activity**

1 In pairs, each take hold of one end of the stick lightly in fingers.
2 Each leading and following, explore where and how the stick can move. Explore the space between each other. Do not allow the stick to fall.

■ **Supplementary development of activity**

Develop to using two sticks.

■ **Additional outcomes**

1 Development of restraining flow focused in the space.
2 Development of sensitivity and sense of lightness.

DEVELOPMENT OF THEME

CARRY

Aims: To support one another in the group, teach lifting strategies
Population: All
Conditions: Trust
Time: 10–15 minutes
Equipment: Possibly a large, strong piece of material for lifters to hold person in
Structure: Groups of five, seven or nine

■ Activity

1 In groups; each group supports fully the weight of one member. Lifters ensure hands are under person's shoulders, hips, head and knees; lifters link arms and bend knees.
2 Progress to carrying the member around the room.
3 Progress to lifting them above heads.

■ Supplementary development of activity

1 Lifters could use material for carrying.
2 Progress to swaying or swinging each member.
3 As a group, give a ride to the person by pulling them along the floor in the material.

■ Additional outcomes

1 Co-operation.
2 Letting go in a group.
3 Trust.

BODY CONTROL 7

Aims: To reduce impulsivity and promote spatial co-ordination

Population: Children, adults

Conditions: None

Time: 2 minutes

Equipment: None

Structure: Whole group

■ Activity

1 Suggest the group walk very fast around the edge of the space in the same direction.
2 Ask them to spiral slowly inwards until centre of space is reached, coming to a stop on arrival.
3 Gradually spiral out again.
4 Repeat inwards spiral and finish in cluster at centre in stillness, then face the walls and walk away from group.
5 Repeat 1–4, but running instead of walking.

■ Additional outcomes

Working as a group in movement and space.

BODY CONTROL 8

Aims: Physical control and development of strength
Population: All
Conditions: None
Time: 2–3 minutes
Equipment: Rhythmical music
Structure: Individual

■ Activity

1 Group copy leader demonstrating raising one leg slowly in standing position (use chair if required at first).
2 Change directions of leg raise, e.g. forward, to one side, behind.
3 Repeat in prone position.

LEVEL 4

Aims: To promote wider vocabulary of movement and adaptation of movements to different levels (see Glossary)
Population: Children
Conditions: None
Time: 2–3 minutes
Equipment: None
Structure: Individually

■ Activity

1   Leader suggests the upper part of the body is opened and stretched at a specific level (see Glossary); for example, stretching out arms horizontally while standing would be a stretch at the medium level.
2   Repeat this opening movement with the upper body but at another level; for example, the same stretch as above while lying down.
3   Now close and curl the upper part of the body at a specified level.
4   Repeat this closing movement at another level.

■ Supplementary development of activity

1   Close upper and open lower part of the body, each at different levels, for example twist and hug the upper body while standing with feet wide apart.
2   Open upper and close lower part of the body, each at different levels.

■ Additional outcomes

Co-ordination between upper and lower parts of the body.

See p. 215 for this activity used in another stage.

TENSION-RELAXATION 4

Aims: To reduce impulsivity and increase control
Population: All
Conditions: None
Time: 5–10 minutes
Equipment: Drum
Structure: Whole group

■ Activity

1 Leader suggests they make a fist, clenching it to the count of 1–5.
2 Reverse count for release of fist and relaxation.
3 Shake out hand and arm.
4 Repeat on other side.

■ Supplementary development of activity

1 Repeat above to drum beats (increase and decrease intensity of sound).
2 Repeat with the jaw area and other muscle groups.

■ Additional outcomes

Isolation of areas of body.

TENSION-RELAXATION 5

Aims: To relax group and separate for closure
Population: All
Conditions: None
Time: 4 minutes
Equipment: None
Structure: Individual

■ **Activity**

1   All lying on backs on mats.
2   Suggest they close eyes and allow body to sink into floor heavily. Picture a blank white screen.
3   Imagine the sun warmly relaxing body, and the floor softly receiving body's weight.
4   Breathe out slowly four times; roll onto left side and wait. Open eyes slowly. Get up in own time.

TENSION-RELAXATION 6

Aim: To close group in manner whereby each is able to leave as an individual
Population: All
Conditions: None
Time: 2 minutes
Equipment: None
Structure: Individual

■ Activity

1 Lie on floor with legs vertically against wall. Ensure base of spine is close to base of wall.
2 Slowly allow legs to open with their own weight, arms behind head.
3 Stay there and be aware of breath for 30 seconds or so.
4 Gently bring legs together, roll onto side and stand up.

■ Additional outcomes

Endurance, inner body sensation, letting go, self-limits, self-trust.

TENSION-RELAXATION 7

Aims: To control and release muscle groups to promote relaxation
Population: All
Conditions: None
Time: 5–10 minutes
Equipment: Mats
Structure: Individual

■ Activity

1 Group lie on backs on mats with open postures.
2 Leader suggests they close eyes, breathe out slowly three times, and respond to suggestions to tighten and relax muscles.
3 Go through areas of body from head to feet, suggesting main muscle groups (and smaller muscle groups if desired).
4 Leader selects participant's head, legs and arms to lift and test on a scale of tension–relaxation.

TENSION-RELAXATION 8

Aim: To close the group
Population: All
Conditions: None
Time: Open-ended
Equipment: None
Structure: Individual

■ **Activity**

1 Lean back against wall in a sitting position on an imaginary seat.
2 Hold position, using tension in thighs, legs, abdominals.
3 See how long the position can be sustained.
4 Move away slowly from wall and shake out legs.

■ **Additional outcomes**

Endurance, inner body sensation, self-limits.

TENSION–RELAXATION 9

Aim: To close the group
Population: All
Conditions: None
Time: 2 minutes
Equipment: None
Structure: Individual

■ Activity

1   Move like a puppet on a string.
2   Move as though held and then flop as if dropped.
3   Move as though held again.

TENSION-RELAXATION 10

Aim: To close the group
Population: All
Conditions: None
Time: 2 minutes
Equipment: None
Structure: Whole group

■ **Activity**

1 Spread fingers of one hand wide and then relax them.
2 Repeat with both hands.
3 Repeat with alternate hands.

FLOOR PATTERN 2

Aims: To experience leading and following as a linked group

Population: Adults, children

Conditions: None

Time: 3–4 minutes

Equipment: None

Structure: Whole group

■ Activity

1   The group make a line holding hands. Designate one of the people on the end as leader.
2   For one minute they walk, twisting and coiling like a snake, following the leader around the space.
3   Reverse this sequence of movements as near as possible, following the person at the other end of line as the leader.
4   Repeat with a new leader and a different method of travel, for example zigzagging.
5   Ask for a volunteer, who then separates from the group.
6   The group continue but make their line into a knot, travelling around and under each other; when thoroughly knotted they freeze, but at no time unclasp hands.
7   The volunteer then attempts to untie the knot by physically manoeuvring the group.

■ Supplementary development of activity

1   Volunteer undoes knot by giving verbal instructions only to group.
2   Group undo own knot non-verbally.

■ Additional outcomes

Physical contact is engendered.

See p.122 for this activity used in another stage.

BODY SENSATION 2

Aims: To become more aware of the tension in our bodies; to begin to release tension
Population: All
Conditions: None
Time: 5 minutes
Equipment: Drum
Structure: Individual

■ Activity

1 While lying on the floor in open position, let eyes close.
2 Leader talks through a count of 1 to 5, during which each member tenses their whole body, including face, and holds breath.
3 Count down from 5 to 1 and release tension built up.
4 Count down from 5 to 1 again for further release using breath.
5 Repeat the above for specific body parts identified by group member.

■ Supplementary development of activity

1 Use drum for build-up of tension; build up slowly in a crescendo.
2 Tension could be expressed in contraction, extension or twisting of body.

■ Additional outcomes

Sense of the tension required and of excessive habitual tension that needs release. Quiet time can enable deep awareness of body.

See p.107 for this activity used in another stage.

MASSAGE

Aims: To warm self and group; relaxation of muscles after physical exertion
Population: All
Conditions: None
Time: 5–10 minutes
Equipment: None
Structure: Whole group

■ Activity

1 Make a close circle, sitting or standing; one behind gently massages the shoulders of one in front.
2 Turn around and repeat.
3 Each to give feedback on how soft/hard they want massage.

See pp.134, 177, 179 and 270 for this activity used in another stage.

STRETCH 1

Aims: To identify and move body parts and muscle groups
Population: All
Conditions: Each session
Time: 5 minutes
Equipment: Music or percussion
Structure: Individual, pairs

■ Activity

1 Leader verbally identifies body parts in turn, and encourages a gradual stretch and release for each named part.
2 Change the levels for stretching, e.g. lying, sitting.
3 Use accompaniment if desired.

■ Supplementary development of activity

Partner B stretches A's limbs gently while lying on floor.

■ Additional outcomes

Awareness of sensation and articulation in body.

See p.132 for this activity used in another stage.

WARM-DOWN

GROUP MOVEMENT

Aim: To let go of left-overs and session work
Population: All
Conditions: Ending a session quietly
Time: 5 minutes
Equipment: Music
Structure: Whole group

■ **Activity**

1 Standing in a circle, in turn lead a movement and say which part you are moving (or leader can specify).
2 Next person in circle moves with a movement that follows on logically.
3 Continue until all group have led movement.

RELATIONSHIP 14

Aim: To wait for turn
Population: All
Conditions: None
Time: Variable
Equipment: None
Structure: Whole group

■ Activity

Whispers with specific actions (e.g. pass on the squeeze) suggested by leader. Action goes around a circle/down a line until it reaches leader again.

RELATIONSHIP 15

Aims: To ground and care for one another in the group
Population: All
Conditions: None
Time: 3–6 minutes
Equipment: Soft music
Structure: Pairs

■ Activity

1 Sitting in pairs, one cradles partner in arms and legs and gives a caring rock.
2 Change over.

■ Additional outcomes

Caring and sensitivity towards others.

BODY BOUNDARY 9

Aim: Differentiation from the environment
Population: All
Conditions: None
Time: 5 minutes
Equipment: None
Structure: Individual

■ Activity

1 All lying relaxed on the floor, prone.
2 Press a named body part that is in contact with the floor down further towards the floor.
3 Use breath; on outbreath make the small movement towards the floor.
4 Work systematically through the whole body.
5 Finish with a slow whole body roll.
6 Notice the body in contact with the floor in the roll.
7 Find a way of standing, being aware of the parts as they leave contact with the floor and those that remain in contact.

■ Supplementary development of activity

1 Press parts against each other, e.g. hand to hand.
2 Press parts against a wall.
3 Press parts against a partner.

■ Additional outcomes

Awareness of own limits, grounding the energy, relationship of body self to the environment.

BODY BOUNDARY 6

Aim: To let go enough to experience self and others
Population: Adults
Conditions: Middle to end of sessions
Time: 5 minutes
Equipment: None
Structure: Individual, pairs

■ Activity

1   Give yourself a hug while sitting down.
2   Repeat standing.
3   Give another group member a hug in the same manner
    as you gave yourself one.
4   Tell them how you experienced their hug.
5   Any ideas about how you took care of yourself?

■ Supplementary development of activity

Hug each member of the group in turn.

■ Additional outcomes

An increased sense of self.Through this physical contact
some issues may arise concerning their experiences of
being held or touched when an infant/child.There may be
an opening up to self-care and to caring for others.

See p. 272 for this activity used in another stage.

BREATH 7

Aim: To focus on exhalation in one part of body
Population: All
Conditions: None
Time: 4–5 minutes
Equipment: None
Structure: Pairs

■ Activity

1 Find a partner.
2 One sits with eyes closed and focuses on breathing out into the open hand of the partner.
3 Their partner places open hand on different areas of abdomen, chest, sides, back and when they feel the breath movement into their hand changes positioning to a different area on upper body.
4 Reverse roles.

■ Additional outcomes

1 Quietening and focusing.
2 Sensitivity towards partner's touch.

BREATH 8

Aim: To promote sense of control
Population: All
Conditions: None
Time: 1–2 minutes
Equipment: None
Structure: Individuals

■ Activity

1 In a circle, sitting, hold one nostril closed and breathe in and out through the other, slowly.
2 Reverse, other nostril held.

INFORMATION

United States

Master's programmes

Antioch University, Keene, NH
40 Avon Street, Keene, NH 03431-3516
Telephone: 603-283-2137
Website: www.antiochne.edu/applied-psychology/dance-movement-therapy/
Contact: admission@antiochcollege.edu
Master's Program in Dance/Movement Therapy and Counseling, Department of Applied Psychology.

Drexel University, Philadelphia, PA
Mail Stop 7905, Three Parkway, 7th Floor, Suite 7103, 1601 Cherry Street, Philadelphia, PA 19102
Telephone: 267-359-5511
Website: http://drexel.edu/cnhp/academics/graduate/MA-Dance-Movement-Therapy-Counseling/
Contact: Kristen Scatton, Dept. Recruitment: kristen.scatton@drexel.edu
MA Dance/Movement Therapy and Counseling, Creative Arts Therapies Department.

Lesley University, Cambridge, MA
29 Everett Street, Cambridge, MA 02138
Telephone: 617-349-8413
Website: www.lesley.edu/master-of-arts/expressive-therapies/dance-therapy/mental-health-counseling/
Contact: Nancy Beardall: beardall@lesley.edu
MA in Clinical Mental Health Counseling: Specialization Dance/Movement Therapy

Naropa University, Boulder, CO
2130 Arapahoe Avenue, Boulder, CO 80302-6697
Telephone: 303-546-3572 and 800-772-6951

Website: www.naropa.edu/academics/masters/clinical-mental-health-counseling/somatic-counseling/dance-move ment-therapy/index.php
Contact: Stephanie San German, Admissions: ssanger-man@naropa.edu
Master of Arts in Clinical Mental Health Counseling, Concentration in Somatic Counseling: Dance/Movement Therapy

Pratt Institute, Brooklyn, NY
200 Willoughby Avenue, Brooklyn NY 11205
Telephone: 718-399-4274
Website: www.pratt.edu/academics/school-of-art/graduate-school-of-art/creative-arts-therapy/creative-arts-therapy-degrees/dance-movement-therapy-ms/
Contact: Joan Wittig, Assistant Professor: jwittig@pratt.edu
Master of Science in Dance/Movement Therapy, Creative Arts Therapy Department

Sarah Lawrence College, Bronxville, NY
1 Mead Way, Bronxville, NY 10708
Telephone: 914-395-2371
Website: www.sarahlawrence.edu/dance-movement-therapy/ #.TxnU6bNnV6c.email
Contact: Jennifer Lemiech-Iervolino, Coordinator: jlemie-chiervolino@sarahlawrence.edu
Emanuel Lomax, Graduate Admissions: elomax@sarahlawr-ence.edu
MSc Degree Program in Dance/Movement Therapy

Doctoral programmes
Drexel University, Philadelphia, PA
1601 Cherry Street, Mail Stop 7905, Philadelphia, PA 19102
Website: http://drexel.edu/cnhp/academics/doctoral/PHD-Creative-Arts-Therapies/
Contacts: Nancy Gerber, Director, PhD Program in Creative Arts Therapies:
ng27@drexel.edu or 267-359-5502

Kristen Scatton, Admissions Coordinator, Department of Creative Arts Therapies: kristen.scatton@drexel.edu or 267-359-5511
Creative Arts Therapies PhD Program, College of Nursing and Health Professions, Drexel University

Lesley University
29 Everett Street, Cambridge, MA 02138
Telephone: 617-349-8166
Website: https://lesley.edu/academics/graduate/expressive-therapies-phd
Contact: Michele Forinash, DA, MT-BC, Director, Expressive Therapies PhD Program: forinasm@lesley.edu
Low residency PhD Program, Expressive Therapies Division, Graduate School of Arts and Social Sciences

Non-academic programmes

Ways of Seeing International Training Program Webinar offered through Dancing Dialogue LCAT, LMHC PLLC
Duration: 2 year/4 semester program
Contact: Dr Suzi Tortora: suzi@suzitortora.com
Website: www.suzitortora.com/ways-of-seeing-international-webinar
Award provided: 8 credits, American Dance Therapy Association Alternate Route DMT training; 30 credits Continuing Education (CE) units American Dance Therapy Association for DMTs

Alternate route programmes

Information for alternate route can be found at: https://adta.org/alternate-route-training/

Europe: all programmes

Germany

Academic programmes

SRH University Heidelberg
Maria-Probst-Str. 3, 69123 Heidelberg, Germany
Faculty of Therapy Sciences, Creative Arts Therapies
MA in Dance Movement Therapy (German and English study track)
Prof. Dr. Douglas R. Keith
Professor
Coordinator of the English tracks: Music Therapy (MA) and Dance Movement Therapy (MA)
Fakultät für Therapiewissenschaften (School of Therapeutic Sciences)
Room E.37a
Maria-Probst-Straße 3
69123 Heidelberg
+49 6221 8223-051
https://www.hochschule-heidelberg.de/en/academics/masterstudium/dance-movement-therapy/

Non-academic programmes

Dance Therapy Centre Berlin
Berlin, Germany
Certificate Dance/Movement Therapist
Imke Fiedler, BC-DMT
www.tanztherapie-zentrum-berlin.de
tanztherapie.zb@t-online.de

European Center for Dance Therapy (Ezetthera)
Munich, Germany
Certified Dance Therapist BTD (equals European MA)
Susanne Bender
www.tanztherapie-zentrum.eu
info@tanztherapie-zentrum.eu

Frankfurt Institute for Dance Therapy
Frankfurt am Main, Germany
Certified Dance/Movement Therapist
www.tanztherapie-fitt.de
info@tanztherapie-fitt.de

German Academy for Psychodynamic Dance Therapy and Expressive Therapy
Bonn, Germany
Dance Therapist and Expressive Therapist Certified DITAT
Dr Sabine Trautmann-Voigt, ADTR
www.tanztherapie.de

Hamburg Institute for Gestalt Oriented Education
Hamburg, Germany
Certificate Dance/Movement Therapist
Inge Matties
www.higw.de
info@higw.de

International Institute for Dance Therapy (IIDT)
Tenerife/Canary Islands (Spain) & Germany
Certificate Dance Therapist BTD & Teacher for the 'Dance of Life'
Petra Klein, Psychologist and Dance Therapist BTD
www.dancetherapy.com, www.tanztherapie.com, www.danzaterapia.com, www.Jardin-Mariposa.com

Langen Institute
Düsseldorf, Germany
Dance/Movement Therapist
Martina Piff
www.langen-institut.de
angen-institut@praeha.de

Pantarhei-Institute for Therapy, Interaction and Dance
Friedland/Göttingen, Germany
Certificate Dance/Movement Therapist

Thomas Wetzorke
www.pantarhei-institut.de
info@pantarhei-institut.de

Psychological Dance Therapy
Hamburg, Germany
Psychotherapeutische Tanztherapeutin
www.pitth.de
pohlmann@pitth.de

Italy

Art Therapy Italiana
Associazione Art Therapy Italiana
Dott.ssa Piera Pieraccini
Bologna—Via Barberia, 13-40123
Roma—c/o Art Therapy Studio—Via Flaminio Ponzio, 18-00145
Firenze—Via San Gallo 79-50129
Torino—Viale Curreno, 41
Milano—Piazzale Baiamonti, 2-20154
051 6440451
Bologna, Roma, Firenze, Torino, Milano
associazione@arttherapyit.org
www.arttherapyit.org

Formazione Triennale in Danzaterapia Clinica VITT3
Lyceum Formazione e Agglornamento
Dott.ssa Laura Pezzenati
Milano, Via Carlo Vittadini, 3
02 36553846-338 2236684
formazione@arteterapia.info
www.arteterapia.info

Scuola Di Arti Terapie
Associazione 'Scuola di Arti Terapie'
Dott. Vincenzo Bellia
Roma

Via Costantino, 41-00145
Catania
Via San Michele, 4-95131
339 1784620-06 40802272
329 6639960

Scuola Di Danzamovimentoterapia Del Centro Di Formazione Nelle Artiterapie Di Lecco
Centro Artiterapie
Dott.a Annapaola Lovisolo
Via Lorenzo Balicco, 11, Lecco, LC, Italia
0341 350496
0341 285012
info@artiterapie.it
www.artiterapie.it/index.php/sections/la-scuola-di-danzamovimentoterapia/

Scuola Di Formazione in Danzamovimentoterapia Dei Processi Evolutivi Psico-Corporei
ARDEIDAE Associazione per la ricerca e lo studio della danzamovimentoterapia e delle tecniche a mediazione corporea
Dott.ssa Daniela Di Mauro
Palermo, piazza Europa, 13
327 1684824
info@associazioneardeidae.org
www.associazioneardeidae.org

Scuola di formazione per operatori in danzaterapia 'm. Fux' e specializzazione in Dmt chiave simbolica ®
Centro Toscano di Arte e Danza Terapia
Dott.ssa Paola De Vera D'Aragona
Firenze—Borgo degli Albizi, 16-50122
055 243008
Firenze
info@centrotoscanodanzaterapia.it
www.centrotoscanodanzaterapia.it

Scuola Di Formazione Professionale in Danzamovimento Terapia Integrata
Coop. Soc. Centro Studi Danza Animazione Arte Terapia
Dott. Vincenzo Puxeddu
Cagliari—via Principe Amedeo, 13
070 650349/665967
Cagliari, Milano, Palermo, Roma
csdanza@tin.it
www.danzamovimentoterapia.it

Scuola Di Formazione Professionale in DMT Espressiva e Psicodinamica
Genova Associazione MetamorfoSidanza
Dr.ssa Cinzia Saccorotti
Sede principale di Genova Associazione MetamorfoSidanza
333694860
cinzia.saccorotti@libero.it
info@metamorfosidanza.com
www.metamorfosidanza.com

Scuola Di Pedagogia Della Mediazione Corporea Ed Espressiva Ad Indirizzo Simbolico-Antropologico
Ass.ne Culturale Eurinome A.S.D.-Perugia
Prof.ssa Alba G. A. Naccari
Sede di Perugia: Via dei Narcisi 41/A 06126-Perugia
Sede di Palmi (RC): Via Virgilio n°78 cap. 89015
338 3442140
alnacc@tin.it
ambrarospo@yahoo.it
www.danzasimbolica.altervista.org

Scuola Di Specializzazione Afgp-Sarabanda in DMT, DMT TRA Oriente Ed Occidente e Metodo Fux. Tecniche e Metodiche Espressive Per Interventi Nel Sociale
Centro Formazione Professionale AFGP-Sarabanda, accreditato dalla Regione Lombardia
Elena Cerruto
Milano—Via Pusiano 52 20123 (MM2 CIMIANO)

02 89404056, 339 2910117
info@associazionesarabanda.it
elenacerruto@gmail.com
www.associazionesarabanda.it

Scuola DMT 'Maria Fux' Centro Risvegli
Scuola DMT 'Maria Fux' Centro Risvegli
Dr. Pietro Farneti
Milano, Italia, via Ventura, 4
0283241125
0232066746
risvegli@fastwebnet.it

Scuola Formazione Professionale DMT Gestalt
Centro Metafora Gestalt Genova
Dott.ssa Mafalda Traveni Massella
Genova—Via Trento, 20/10-16145
010 364955
010 3107147
danzaterapia@metaforagestalt.it

Europe: *academic programmes*

Belgium

Agape
Located in Koolskamp
4-year dance movement therapy training, which leads to a certificate.
Programme is approved by BVCT-ABAT.
www.agapebelgium.be

Artevelde University College
Advanced Bachelor degree, Arts Therapies (incorporating art therapy, dance movement therapy, dramatherapy or music therapy).
Part-time programme consisting of 6 modules.

Estonia

Tallin University
Creative Arts Therapies Program
Two-year Master's Program
Dance Movement Therapy, School of Natural Sciences and Health

France

University Sorbonne, Paris
MA Professional and Research in Artistic Creation
Specialization in Dance Therapy
Contact: Prof. Todd Lubart
Université Paris Descartes/Sorbonne Paris Cité
Institut de Psychologie
Scolarité Master
71 avenue Edouard Vaillant
921090 Boulogne Billancourt
scol-master-creation-artistique@psychologie.parisdes-cartes.fr
www.parisdescartes.fr

Hungary

Training Institute of Hungarian Association for Movement and Dance Therapy Psychodynamic Movement and Dance Therapy (PMDT)
6 years (12 semesters) of training
www.tancterapia.net/kepzes_pdmt.htm

Latvia

Stradins University Riga
Medical School
MA in Healthcare, Art Therapy specialization Dance Movement Therapy
www.dkt.lv/en/

The Netherlands

Inspirees Dance Movement Therapy Training
Certificate and American Dance Therapy Association alternate route to registration
Europe
A v Scheltemaplein
2624PJ, Delft
The Netherlands
+31 (0)15 8795501
Contact: Nuo Yang +31 (0)64744 5687

Nijmegen: Han University of Applied Sciences (Han)
Bachelor of Arts (art, drama, music, or psychomotor therapy)
Hogeschool van Arnhem en Nijmegen
Institute of Art Therapies, Psychomotor Therapy and Applied Psychology
Postbus 6960
6503 GL, Nijmegen, NL
Tel: +31 648382329
www.han.nl
robert.vandenbroek@han.nl

Rotterdam Dance Academy
Kruisplein 26. 3012 CC Rotterdam
Tel: +31 (0)10 2171100
Contact (Coordinator): N. Wentholt
Department of Codarts, University of Professional Arts Education. Master's in Dance Therapy—2 year part-time programme taught in English.
www.codarts.nl/pragrammes/dance/dancetherapy/

Zuyd
Bachelor of Art Therapies Program
www.creatievetherapie.hsz.nl/
0031 (0)464006330

Poland

Polish Institute for Dance Movement Psychotherapy
4-year postgraduate training in Dance Movement Psychotherapy
Diploma of completion
www.instytutdmt.pl

Russia

Institute of Practical Psychology and Psychoanalysis
Dance Movement Psychotherapy Post Graduate Professional Training (3 years)
tdt-edu.ru/programs/tancevalno-dvigatelnaya-psixoterapiya/
atda.ru/professionalnoe-obuchenie/tancevalno-dvigatelnaya-psihotherapiya
Director: Irina Biryukova, BC-DMT iradmt@gmail.com
Advisor: Patrizia Pallaro, BC-DMT

Slovenia

University of Ljubljana
MA in Support through the Arts
(Dance Movement Therapy)
2 years, part-time
www.pef.uni-lj.si
alenkavidrih@siol.com
++386 1 429 32 00

Spain

Autonomous University of Barcelona
Coordination: Heidrun Panhofer, Assumpta RatAcs Edifici d'Estudiants (R) PlaAa CAvica Campus de Bellaterra
Tel: 93 581 2990
Fax: 93 581 3099
Contact: master.dmt@uab.es
Master and Postgraduate Diploma in DMT

Switzerland

Institute for Dance Therapy at the Lake
CH 8593 Kesswil, Switzerland
Ana Bella Nosa-Quaas
www.tanztherapie-am-see.ch
infor@tanztherapie-am-see.ch

UK

Goldsmiths College, University of London
MA Dance Movement Psychotherapy
Caroline Frizell
c.frizell@gold.ac.uk
www.gold.ac.uk/pg/ma-dance-movement-psychotherapy/

University of Derby
MA Dance Movement Psychotherapy
Dr Jill Bunce
j.bunce@derby.ac.uk
www.derby.ac.uk/courses/postgraduate/dance-movement-psychotherapy-ma/

University of Roehampton
MA Dance Movement Psychotherapy
Dr Beatrice Allegranti
b.allegranti@goehampton.ac.uk
www.roehampton.ac.uk/podance-movement-psy/dance-movement-psychotherapy/index.html

Europe: *doctoral programmes*

UK

University of Hertfordshire
de Havilland Campus,
Hatfield Business Park,
Hatfield,

Hertfordshire
AL10 9EU
Tel: 0044 (0) 1707 285861
Contact: Professor Helen Payne, PhD: H.L.Payne@herts.ac.uk
Doctorate by research in Dance Movement Psychotherapy/ Body Psychotherapy/Arts Therapies
www.herts.ac.uk

University of Roehampton
PhD in All Arts Therapies
Beatrice Allegranti, PhD: b.allegranti@goehampton.ac.uk
www.roehampton.ac.uk/postgraduate-courses/dance-movement-psychotherapy/index.html

Israel

Academic College of Society and the Arts, Israel
(Art Therapy, Psychodrama, Dance Movement)
10b Ha'Orzim Street, P.O. Box 13335, Netanya, 42379
Tel: 011-972-9-8656501
Samuel Schwartz, PhD sschwar@asa.ac.il
www.asa.ac.il/

David Yelin Academic College of Education
(Art Therapy, Dance Movement, Bibliotherapy, Music Therapy)
Ma'agal Beit HaMidrash St 7, Jerusalem
Tel: +972-2-6558111
Orit Sônia Waisman, PhD: orito@dyellin.ac.il
www.dyellin.ac.il/
www.yahat.org/pages/About_us.aspx

Kibbutzim College of Education
(Art Therapy, Psychodrama, Dance Movement, Bibliotherapy)
149 Namir, Tel Aviv 62507
Tel: 036905433
Arts.Therapy@smkb.ac.il

Head of MA Programme: Dr Maya Vulcan
The Creative-Expressive Therapies Training Center

University of Haifa
MA Graduate School of Creative Art Therapies
Training program in DMT
Dita Federman, PhD: ditafederman@gmail.com
Einat Shufer, PhD: einatsh2@bezeqint.net
http://artherapy.haifa.ac.il/index_eng.html
University of Haifa, Israel is launching a new international MA program in creative art therapies (including dance/movement therapy) taught in English. Haifa International.

Asia: non-academic programmes

China

China–Germany Professional Dance Therapy Training, Beijing
Susanne Bender, MA; Weixiao Li, PhD
EZETTHERA—Europaeisches Zentrum fuer Tanztherapie, Germany
Tel: +49/89/54662431
www.tanztherapie-zentrum.eu

Inspirees Dance Movement Therapy Training
Certificate and American Dance Therapy alternate route to registration
Europe
A v Scheltemaplein
2624PJ, Delft
The Netherlands
Tel: +31 (0)15 8795501
Contact: Nuo Yang +31 (0)64744 5687
China
Ocean Express Building F, Xiaguangli 66, 100027, Beijing
+86 (0)10 8446 7947
+86 (0)10 8446 7847

Contact: Katee Shen, 15911509565
Email: dmt@inspirees.com
www.dancetherapy.cn
Blogwww.weibo.com/dancetherapy
Hong Kong
Flat C1, 20/F, Mai On Industrial Bldg, 17–21 Kung Yip St.,
Kwai Chung,
+852 9087 7043
Email: lifeoriginhk@yahoo.com.hk
www.lifeoriginhk.com

India

Creative Movement Therapy Association of India
25-C Prithviraj Road, behind 25-A & near Tata House, New
Delhi—110011
Tel: +91 9819886649
Contact: Reetu Jain: info@cmtai.org; reetu@cmtai.org
www.cmtai.org
Certificate course in DMT in New Delhi and Bangalore

**Kolkata Sanved and the Center for Lifelong Learning,
Tata Institute of Social Sciences, Mubaipostal**
60 Dasnagar, P.D.-Lake Gardens, Kolkata-700045m West
Bengal
Tel: (033) 24993126; Mobile: 09836469932
Contact: Kolkata Sanved: kolkatasanved@gmail.com; Nam-
rata Kanuga
www.kolkatasanved.org
Director: Sohini Chakraborty
Diploma course in DMT of 660 hours

South Korea

**Korean Dance Therapy Association of Arts Therapy
Academy of Korea, South Korea**
269 Changgyeonggung-ro, Jongno-gu, Seoul
Tel: 82-2-744-5157

Fax: 82-2-744-5159
Boon Soon Ryu, PhD
kdmta@naver.com
www.kdmta.com/eng/
2-year training programme to prepare a dance therapist

Asia: academic programmes

South Korea

Seoul Women's University Graduate School of Professional Therapeutic Technology
Tel: 82-2-970-5887
Na Yung Kim, PhD: nayungkim@swu.ac.kr
www.swu.ac.kr/special/eng/new/en_about_01.html
Master's and PhD degree in DMT major of Expressive Arts Therapy Department

Soon Chun Hyang University Graduate School of Psychotherapy Department
Major in Dance Therapy
22, Soonchunhyang-ro, Sinchang-myeon, Asan-si, Chungcheongnam-do
Tel: 82-10-3007-9682
Boon Soon Ryu, PhD: kdmta@naver.com
https://homepage.sch.ac.kr/egradu/02/03.jsp
3-year training program, MA and PhD degrees major in Dance Therapy, Department of Psychotherapy

Australia

International Dance Therapy Institute
P.O. Box 5168, Mordialloc,
Victoria 3195
Tel: 61-439 330 008
admin@idtia.org.au
www.idtia.org.au

The University of Melbourne
Creative Arts Therapies Research Unit,
Building 862,
234 St Kilda Road,
Southbank,
Victoria 3006
Contact: Dr Kim Dunphy: k.dunphy@unimelb.edu.au
https://finearts-music.unimelb.edu.au/research/our-research/creative-arts-therapies-research-unit
PhD Program, Creative Arts and Music Therapy Research Group
Masters Creative Arts Therapies in development stage—Dance Movement/Drama Therapies

South America

Argentina

Brecha Energia Movimiento Cambio
Quesada 3470. (1430) Buenos Aires, Argentina
Tel: 541/542-4623
Diana Fischman, PhD: dfischman@brecha.com.ar
DMT Argentina Training Program includes BC-DMT trainers

Caece University
Buenos Aires
Tel: 54/1 52522812 or 43/1 48070828
eroisen@caece.edu.ar
Maralia Reca, PhD, reca.maralia@gmail.com
Postgraduate training program in DMT

UNA: Universidad Nacional de las Artes
movimiento.una.edu.ar
Sánchez de Loria 443
Ciudad Autónoma de Buenos Aires
Tel: (+54.11) 4866.2168
https://movimiento.una.edu.ar/carreras/maestria-en-danza-movimiento-terapia_16729

DANCE MOVEMENT THERAPY PROFESSIONAL ASSOCIATIONS

The American Dance Therapy Association, Suite 108, 2000 Century Plaza, 10632 Little Patuxent Parkway, Columbia, Maryland 21044, USA, www.adta.org

Arts Therapies Professional Associations (UK)
Association of Professional Music Therapists, www.bamt.org.uk
British Association of Art Therapists, www.baat.org.uk
British Association of Dramatherapists, www.badth.org.uk

The Association for Dance Movement Therapy, Spain
www.danzamovimientoterapia.com/
admte@danzamovimientoterapia.com

The Association for Dance Movement Psychotherapy, UK, 22 Church Road, Weston, Bath BA1 4BT. Publishes quarterly newsletter, organises monthly workshops and Summer schools, publications, support groups, network. admin@admp.org.uk www.admp.org.uk

Czech Dance and Movement Therapy Association (TANTER)
www.arttherapies.cz/eng/the-czech-dance-and-movement-therapy-association.html
beatealbrich@seznam.cz

European Association for Dance Movement Therapy
www.eadmt.com
info@eadmt.com

Dance Movement Therapy Association, Russia
www.atdt.ru/desc_text.php?menu=english
tdtatdt@mail.ru

German Professional Organisation for Dance Therapists
www.btd-tanztherapie.de/BTDengl/_E_index.htm
info@BTD-taztherapie.de

Greek Association of Dance Therapists
http://gadt.gr/english.htm
dancetherapy@gadt.gr

Hungarian Association for Dance Movement Therapy
http://mozgasterapia.net/
konferencia@tancterapia.net

Israeli Association for Creative Arts Therapies (Yahat)
www.yahat.org/pages/About_us.aspx

Latvian Dance Movement Therapy Association
http://dkt.lv/en/
dkt.valde@gmail.com

The Netherlands Association for Dance Movement Therapy
www.nvdat.nl/
nvdat.info@vaktherapie.nl

Professional Association of Dance Movement Therapy, Italy
www.apid.it/info.htm
segreteria@apid.it

Swedish Association of Dance Therapy
www.dansterapi.info
styrelsen@dansterapi.info

UK Psychotherapy Professional Organisations and Training

Association for Humanistic Psychology Practitioners, Member organisation HIPC UKCP www.ahpp.org.uk
British Association for Counselling and Psychotherapy
www.bacp.co.uk
British Psychotherapy Foundation
www.britishpsychotherapyfoundation.org.uk
Gestalt Centre, Training in Gestalt Psychotherapy. Supervision
www.gestaltcentre.co.uk

Guild of Psychotherapists
www.guildofpsychotherapists.org.uk
Institute of Group Analysis, Training and therapy
www.groupanalysis.org
Lincoln Clinic and Institute for Psychotherapy, Training and therapy
www.lincoln-psychotherapy.org.uk
Metanoia, Psychotherapy Training Institute, Supervision and training www.metanoia.ac.uk
Minster Centre, Psychotherapy training
www.minstercentre.ac.uk
Re-vision, Psychosynthesis and Education Trust, (psycho-synthesis/transpersonal) Training www.re-vision.org.uk
Society of Analytical Psychology (Jungian)
www.thesap.org.ukThe Tavistock Institute of Human Relations, Training
www.tavinstitute.org.uk
United Kingdom Council for Psychotherapy
www.psychotherapy.org.uk

Other relevant organisations

Arts for Health, Royal Society for Public Health
www.rsph.org.uk/our-work/policy/wellbeing/arts-and-health.html
Laban Guild, Workshops in the Laban approach
www.labanguild.org.uk
London Centre for Psychodrama, Training and supervision
www.londoncentreforpsychodrama.org.uk

GLOSSARY OF TERMS

Asymmetry Where one side of the body moves in a different manner from the other.

Body boundary   That physical entity from which all perception is recorded and expressed.

Body image   The psycho-emotional sense we have of our bodies, related to self-image, formed both by others' feedback to us about our bodies and by our own perception of our bodies.

Body shape   The body has a natural capacity to stretch, twist and bend, resulting in shapes that can be, for example, flat, pointed, crooked or rounded.

Centring   There is a feeling of balance and inner strength when we are centred. To feel centred is to experience one's psychological centre of gravity, felt in the solar plexus. (See Hendricks and Wills, 1975.)

Diagonals   These are combinations of left/right and backward/forward (e.g. right forward) with levels high and low. For example, left forward high to right backward low, or vice versa; both possible with each side of the body leading the movement.

Dimensions of space   When we move in a direction (left/right/forward/backward) and also in a high or low level, dimensions are the result. These lead to movements of closing and opening, advancing and retreating, rising and sinking.

Grounding   A basic trust of one's body and a sound relationship to gravity. Misuse of or interference with our essential natures leads to frustration and dissatisfied separation from our bodily ground. (See Keleman, 1981.)

Levels   Three levels, high, medium and low. High is the furthest point one can reach from the joint from which the movement is activated in gesture (e.g. with arms or legs). Medium level is when, e.g. the leg is used at hip level, high when it is above the hips, and low when below the hips. With the arm the reference point is the shoulder. The action of stepping would be high if on the toes, medium if on whole sole of foot, and low if done with bent knees.

Locomotion   *See travelling.*

Pathways We can move in straight, angular or twisted ways in our own personal space, creating different patterns, whether with whole body or gestures of arms, legs etc. These pathways are in the air around us, in general space. Moving over the floor we also create patterns in straight, angular or twisted pathways, which create a floor pattern.

Perseveration Repetitive movement that leads nowhere, e.g. turning a tap on and off. Often found in disturbed clients.

Populations This refers to the client groups that may be found in need of special care and intervention, for example, the learning disabled or psychiatric populations.

Re-birthing Re-birthing itself is seen as a spiritual discipline where the birth experience is re-lived. Sometimes the process of initiating the birthing movement patterns triggers deeply repressed birth memories and re-activates the primal struggle to live or die. Primal therapy in particular can assist in integrating these experiences.

Relationship This implies initiating, maintaining, rejecting or ignoring contact. It involves listening, watching or responding to contact, whether visual, verbal, tactile, kinaesthetic or auditory, with others, objects, or the space.

Ritual An often-repeated series of actions; a performance of rites; a body or code of ceremonies. This could be, for example, the group's agreed and intentional convention, such as how the session starts and finishes.

Symmetry Movement where both sides of the body move in the same manner/shape at the same time.

Travelling/locomotion Form of stepping in general space. Going from one place to another in a transference of weight.

Under-bounded Where the individual is lacking in containment; much free flow of movement as in hyperactivity or flaccidity.

JOURNALS

International Journal of Body, Movement and Dance in Psychotherapy
An academic journal, four issues per annum, peer reviewed and published by Taylor & Francis
www.tandfonline.com/toc/tbmd20/current

American Dance Therapy Journal
An academic journal, four issues per annum, peer reviewed and published by Elsevier
https://adta.org/american-dance-therapy-journal/

The Arts in Psychotherapy
An academic journal, four issues per annum, peer reviewed and published by Springer
www.sciencedirect.com/journal/the-arts-in-psychotherapy

Creative Arts Therapies
Published by the German Scientific Association of Creative Arts Therapies (http://wfkt.de/)
www.egms.de/static/en/journals/index.htm

Irish Association of Creative Arts Therapies Journal
www.iacat.ie

Creative Arts in Education and Therapy (CAET) www.caet.quotus.org

Dance Research Journal, www.dancestudiesassociation.org/publications/dance-research-journal

RESOURCE BASE

It is useful to develop for yourself a wide repertoire of resources. The following are some suggestions.

Equipment

Little is needed to practice in a 'barefoot' sense, apart from a suitable space. However, the following are useful:

(a) music player;
(b) a selection of music by developing your own playlist (e.g. Spotify: www.spotify.com);
(c) props such as elastic, parachute, material, mats;
(d) percussion instruments;
(e) sheets of drawing paper and felt-tip pens or crayons.

Source books

These books are useful for delving into for further information and materials.

Amans D, *An Introduction to Community Dance Practice*, second edition, Red Globe Press, 2017.

Baldwin F and Whitehead M, *That Way and This (Poetry for Dance)*, London: Chatto & Windus, 1972.

Bartenieff I, 'How Is the Dancing Teacher Equipped to Do Dance Therapy?'. In E Thayer Gaston (Ed.), *Music Therapy*, Lawrence, Kansas: The Allen Press, 1957.

Bartenieff I and Lewis D, *Body Movement: Coping with the Environment*, London: Gordon & Breach Science Publishers, 1980.

Bate R, Weir M and Parker C, *Movement and Growth Programmes for the Elderly and Those Who Care for Them*, London: ADMP Publications, 1985.

Benson JF, *Working more Creatively with Groups*, London: Tavistock, 1987.

Boadella D, *Lifestreams: An Introduction to Biosynthesis*, London: Routledge & Kegan Paul, 1987.

Bond T, *Games for Social and Life Skills*, London: Hutchinson, 1986.

Bowlby J, *The Making and Breaking of Affectional Bonds*, London: Tavistock, 1979.

Bradling R, *Festive Occasions in the Primary School,* London: Ward Lock, 1981.

Brown NW, *Creative Activities for Group Therapy,* London: Routledge, 2013.

Caplow-Lindner E et al., *Therapeutic Dance Movement: Expressive Activities for Older Adults,* New York/London: Human Sciences Press, 1979.

Casement P, *On Learning from the Patient,* London & New York: Tavistock Publications, 1985.

Chaiklin, S (Ed.) *Marian Chace: Her Papers,* Columbia, MD: American Dance Therapy Association, 1975.

Chaiklin S and Wengrower H (Eds.), *The Art and Science of Dance/Movement Therapy: Life is Dance,* London: Routledge, 2009.

Chaiklin S and Wengrower H (Eds.), *The Art and Science of Dance/Movement Therapy: Life is Dance,* second edition, London: Routledge, 2016.

Cheney G and Strader J, *Modern Dance,* Boston, MA: Allyn and Bacon, 1975.

Chesner A and Hahn H (Eds.), *Creative Advances in Group Work,* Philadelphia, PA: Jessica Kingsley Publishers, 2002.

Chesner A and Zografou L, *Creative Supervision across Modalities,* London: Jessica Kingsley Publishers, 2014.

Corrigall J, Payne H and Wilkinson H (Eds.), *About a Body: Working with the Embodied Mind in Psychotherapy,* London: Routledge, 2006.

Costonis MN, *Therapy in Motion,* Chicago, IL: University of Illinois Press, 1978.

Dell C, *A Primer for Movement Description,* New York: Dance Notation Bureau, 1970.

Erikson E, *Childhood and Society,* Harmondsworth: Penguin, 1978.

Ernst S and Goodison L, *In Our Own Hands: A Book of Self-Help Therapy,* London: The Women's Press, 1981.

Feder E and Feder B, *The Expressive Arts Therapies: Art, Music and Dance as Psychotherapy,* New Jersey: Prentice-Hall, 1981.

Ferrucci P, *What We May Be. An Introduction to Psychosynthesis,* Northamptonshire, UK: Turnstone Press, 1982.

Fisher S and Cleveland SE, *Body Image and Personality,* New York, NY: Dover, 1968.

Fraleigh S, *Moving Consciously,* University of Illinois, 2015.

Garcia M, Plevin M and Macagno P, *Creative Movement and Dance,* Rome: Gremese, 2006.

Gellhorn E, 'Motion and Emotion: The Role of Proprioception in the Philosophy and Pathology of the Emotions', *Psychological Review,* 71, pp. 457–472, 1964.

Gendlin E, 'Focusing', *Journal of Psychotherapy, Research and Practice,* 6, pp. 4–15, 1962.

Goodill SW, *An Introduction to Medical Dance/Movement Therapy: Health Care in Motion,* London: Jessica Kingsley Publishers, 2005.

Hanna JL, *To Dance Is Human. A Theory of Non-verbal Communication,* Austin, TX/London: University of Texas Press, 1979.

Harris JG, *A Practicum for Dance Therapy,* London: ADMP Publications, 1984.

Hayes J, *Soul and Spirit in Dance Movement Psychotherapy: A Transpersonal Approach,* Jessica Kingsley Publishers, 2013.

Holle B, *Motor Development in Children: Normal and Retarded,* Oxford: Blackwell Scientific Publications, 1981.

Huang A, *Embrace Tiger, Return to Mountain: The Essence of T'ai Chi,* Moab, UT: Real People Press, 1973.

Jennings S (Ed.), *Creative Therapy,* London: Pitman, 1973.

Jung CG, *Man and His Symbols,* Harmondsworth: Penguin, 1964.

Kakou V and Sanderson P, *Arts Therapies: A Research Based Map of the Field,* Elsevier, 2006.

Kestenberg Amighi J, Loman S, Lewis P and Sossin M, *The Meaning of Movement: Developmental and Clinical Perspectives of the Kestenberg Movement Profile,* London: Routledge, 2014.

Kestenberg J, 'The Role of Movement, Patterns in Development', *Psychoanalytic Quarterly,* 36:3, pp. 356–409, 1967.

Lefco H, *Dance Therapy: Narrative Case Histories of Therapy Sessions with Six Patients*, Chicago, IL: Nelson Hall, 1973.

Leventhal M, *Movement & Growth: Dance Therapy for the Special Child*, New York, NY: New York University Press, 1980.

Levete G, *No Handicap to Dance*, London: Souvenir Press, 1982.

Levy F, *Dance/Movement Therapy: A Healing Art*, NDA/AAHPERD, Virginia, 1988.

Lewis P (Ed.), *Theory and Methods in Dance Movement Therapy*, Iowa: Kendall/Hunt Publishing, 1972.

Lewis P (Ed.), *Theoretical Approaches in Dance Movement Therapy*, vol. 1, Iowa: Kendall/Hunt Publishing, 1979.

Lewis P (Ed.), *Theoretical Approaches in Dance Movement Therapy*, vol. 2, Iowa: Kendall/Hunt Publishing, 1984.

Lowen A, *The Language of the Body*, London: Collier Macmillan, 1971.

Madori LL, *Therapeutic Thematic Arts Programming for Older Adults*, Baltimore, MD: Health Professions Press, 2007.

Mason KC (Ed.), *Focus on Dance VII—Dance Therapy*, Washington DC: American Association of Health, Education & Recreation, 1974.

Mather C, *Building Blocks for Creative Movement*, DVD available: www.sherbornemovementuk.org

McNiff S, *The Arts and Psychotherapy*, Springfield, IL: Charles Thomas, 1981.

Meekums B, *Creative Group Therapy for Women Survivors of Child Sexual Abuse*, London: Jessica Kingsley Publishers, 2000.

Moore CL, *Executives in Action*, Plymouth: Macdonald & Evans, 1982. (1st edn, 1978, entitled *Action Profiling.*)

Newlove J, *Laban for All*, Nick Hearn Books, 2003.

Pallero P (Ed.), *Authentic Movement: Essays by Mary Starks Whitehouse, Janet Adler and Joan Chodorow*, London: Jessica Kingsley Publishers, 1999.

Pallero P (Ed.), *Authentic Movement: Moving the Body, Moving the Self, Being Moved. A Collection of Essays. Volume Two*, London: Jessica Kingsley Publishers, 2007.

Parratt AL, *Indoor Games and Activities*, London: Hodder & Stoughton, 1983.

Payne HL (Ed.), *Supervision of Dance Movement Psychotherapy*, London: Routledge, 2008.

Pierce-Jones F, *The Alexander Technique: Body Awareness in Action*, New York, NY: Schosken Books, 1976.

Preston-Dunlop V, *A Handbook for Modern Educational Dance*, London: Macdonald Evans, 1963.

Rubio R, *Mind/Body Techniques for Asperger's Syndrome*, London: Jessica Kingsley Publishers, 2008.

Sacks O, *The Man Who Mistook His Wife for a Hat*, London: Picador, Pan Books, 1985.

Saltzberger-Wittenberg I, *Psychoanalytic Insight and Relationships*, London: Routledge & Kegan Paul, 1970.

Scheflen AE, with Scheflen A, *Body Language and The Social Order*, Englewood Cliffs, NJ: Prentice-Hall, 1972.

Schilder P, *The Image and Appearance of the Human Body*, New York, NY: International Universities Press, 1955.

Schwartz-Salant N and Stein M (Eds.), *The Body in Analysis*, Illinois: Chiron, 1986.

Sheets-Johnstone M, *The Phenomenology of Dance*, Philadelphia, PA: Temple University Press, 2015.

Shreeves R, *Children Dancing*, London: Ward Lock Educational, 1979.

Silbermann L (Ed.), *Dance Therapy Bibliography*, Columbia, MD: American Dance Therapy Association, 1984.

Spencer P, *Society and the Dance*, Cambridge University Press, 1986.

Stokes EM, *Word Pictures as a Stimulus for Creative Dance*, London: MacDonald & Evans, 1970.

Totton N and Edmondson E, *Reichian Growth Work*, Dorset, UK: Prism Press, 1988.

Tufnell M, *When I Opened My Eyes: Dance Health Imagination*, London: Dance Books, 2017.

Tufnell M and Crickmay C, *A Widening Field: Journeys in Body and Imagination*, Hampshire: Dance Books, 2004.

Tufnell MB and Crickmay C, *Body Space Image*, London: Dance Books, 2014.

Unkovitch J, Butte C and Butler J (Eds.), *Dance Movement Psychotherapy with People with Learning Disabilities*, London: Routledge, 2017.

White T, *Visual Poetry for Creative Interpretation*, London: MacDonald & Evans, 1969.

Wosien M, *Sacred Dance: Encounter with the Gods*, London: Thames and Hudson, 1974.

Zukav G, *The Dancing Wu Li Masters*, London: Fontana, 1979.

Other areas to explore in books could be stories, mythology and science fiction. For background reading on the history of the Arts and Disabilities:

The Attenborough Report (1985), Carnegie UK Trust, Bedford Square Press.

After Attenborough (1988), Carnegie UK Trust, Bedford Square Press.

The use of music for creative dance and movement

First a word about the limitations in using music. One of the greatest problems when using pre-recorded music with your groups is that the movement may need to change in its quality or rhythm, but the music will continue to impose its essential phrasing etc. This could impede the group's creativity and distract from the group development and process. Percussion used by you to reflect, for example, group mood, rhythm and/or process is a good alternative. Music cannot respond to the immediacy of individual and group emotion, although it may be selected purposely to pre-empt, contradict or reflect emotional states present in the group. Some groups may become dependent upon the music, being unable to motivate themselves, with the resulting loss in spontaneity. Familiar music may stimulate past memories and perhaps have specific phenomena associated with it that could negatively or positively influence the group. Music can be too controlling, especially if the leader is the only person in the group to select it. It can also dictate the mood, the rhythm, the movement and the energy level for the group. This may result in a repression or an ignoring of fundamental needs. Although these factors may be entirely appropriate for your group/s and the aims/objectives you have set, you will need to be familiar with the music in your resource bases and to be clear why you are using it. An understanding of music's powerful qualities and its advantages and disadvantages at different stages of your group's life can free you and your group.

The choice of music is very personal. Whatever motivates you to dance is usually a useful guideline. Music may be used in many ways, for example:

1   The dance may follow the construction of music that has a *shaping* emphasis and a repetition of the same theme, e.g. *Monotones* by Erik Satie, or as in a fugue. It may suggest different people moving at different times or different groups of people. One person may follow the theme, whilst others accompany with smaller/bigger variations on their dance movements.
2   The dance could be based on the mood or feeling—the tone of the music—that is, it could be interpreted emotionally, e.g. Bessie Smith 'Blues' songs, *Star Wars* theme tune.
3   The dance could be a reaction to the action and rhythm of the music e.g. Mussorsky *Pictures at an Exhibition*, Gnome section.
4   The music could set an atmosphere for a dance drama, e.g. *Echoes* by Emerson, Lake and Palmer or *War of the Worlds* by Jeff Wayne. The movement will still need

to follow the climax, change, increases and decreases, and pauses in the music, however.

5 Individual instruments may be followed in the dance, giving variety and relationship to a group dance.

When using music for interpretation it is important that the piece be short, especially for those with limited attention spans. Select a piece that you know well enough to fade out at a given place. It could be pre-recorded with a fade. You may need to allow time in the session to rehearse dances without accompaniment.

Music can be used as a stimulus motivator or as an accompaniment for the dance. If working with live musicians, a piece of music can be composed as the dance is made or following the choreography of the piece. Percussion may be used after the dance has been created in a similar manner. Pre-recorded music can also be added afterwards, although the shape of the dance will have to be adapted in places.

Music may be used at any point during the session to accompany warm-up activities, creative work or a completed dance. One piece or two contrasting pieces may be used. It may be good for safety, encouraging movement and relaxing inhibitions, for some groups. Below are a few selections from music (pre-recorded) that have been found to be useful. The list is not intended to be comprehensive.

General

Andrews Sisters—any appropriate
Blue—Otis Reading
Blue Danube—Strauss
Brandenburg Concertos—London Philharmonic Orchestra
Capriccio Espagnol and Scheherazade—Rimsky-Korsakov
Carnival of the Animals—Saint-Saëns
Cavatina/Romanza—John Williams

Ghost Dances—The Mercury Ensemble (South American)
Folk Songs. Arranged Nicholas Carr courtesy of Inti-illimani
Greatest Hits—Paul Simon
Guitar Recital—John Williams
La Flute Indienne—Los Calchakis et Los Gaucharacos
Lord of the Rings—Bo Hanson
On Broadway—George Benson
Piano Rags (The Entertainer)—Scott Joplin
Pictures at an Exhibition—Mussorgsky
Playground on Mars (Chariots of Fire)—Vangelis
Ritual Fire Dance—De Falla
Snowflakes are Dancing—Tomita
Switched on Bach
Toyshop from *The Sorcerer's Apprentice*, Paul Dukas
Variations—Andrew Lloyd Webber
Water Music—Handel

Stepping (warm-up)

Borodin, Palovtsian Dances from Prince Igor—Rimsky-Korsakov and Glazunov
Cacharpaya—Incantations
Dr Who Theme—BBC Records
Favorite Piano Pieces—Chopin, Decca
The Flight of the Condor—BBC Records
Golliwogs' Cakewalk—Mussorgsky
Hall of the Mountain King—Grieg
Jungle Rhythms and Chants—Olympic Records
The Light of Experience—Gheorghe Zamfir
Music from India No. 10—Imrat Kahn
Pizzicato Polka, Circus, Tritsch-Tratsch Polka—Strauss
The Planets Suite—Holst

Light and fun (warm-up)

Bach—any appropriate
Chopin—Any piano pieces

Floral Dance—Brighouse and Rastrick Brass Band
Mikrokosmos—Bartok
Vivaldi—any appropriate

Dreamy blues

Ain't Misbehavin'—Fats Waller (RCA)
Drinking Rum and Coca-Cola—Andrews Sisters
God Bless the Child—Billie Holiday

Step patterns and rhythms

Music of Mikis Theodorikis (Zorba's Dance)
Thriller (The Beat)—Michael Jackson
Tijuana Brass Albums

Stately, regular

Gymnopedies 1, 2 & 3—Erik Satie (from *Monotones*)
Historical Dance Music
Largo—Handel
Pomp and Circumstance—Edward Elgar (*Clockwork Orange*
film theme—Henry Purcell)

Quick and exciting

Baggy Trousers—Madness
National Folk Dance Music

Dramatic (could follow story line)

March of Dwarfs—Grieg, Lyric Suite, Op. 54
Piano Man—Billy Joel

Shaping dances

Begegnungen—Eno, Moebius, Roedelius, Plank
Bolero—Ravel
Fingal's Cave—Mendelssohn
The Good, the Bad and the Ugly (theme)—Morricone
Le Cygne—Saint Saëns

Masters of Irish Music—Martin Byrnes
New World Symphony—Dvorak
Peer Gynt, Morning—Grieg
Prelude à L'Après-Midi d'un Faune—Debussy
World of Mozart—Mozart

Strength and atmosphere

Cantavina—John Williams
Sky—I and II (Ariola Records)
Slip Slidin' Away—Paul Simon

Soft feeling tones

Albatross—Fleetwood Mac
Nocturne Op. 15 no. 2—Chopin
Waltz No. 14—Chopin

You will need to listen to a wide range of music. Remember it is the synthesis of the movement and the music that is exciting, showing the shape of the phrase and the flow of the music. The best way to form ideas and impressions of the use of music is to see other people's approaches to the problem. It is desirable to get to live performances of music and dance as much as possible. All major dance companies have education officers who will inform you of local opportunities for seeing their company perform. There are many companies who see their role as educating in dance as an art form and who will visit your setting for workshops and performances.

REFERENCES

Adler J, *Offering from the Conscious Body: The Discipline of Authentic Movement*, Rochester, VT: Inner Traditions, 2002.

Adrian B, *Actor Training the Laban Way: An Integrated Approach to Voice, Speech, and Movement*, New York: Allworth Press, 2008.

Allport GW, *Pattern and Growth in Personality*, New York: Holt, Rinehart & Winston, 1961.

Bainbridge G, Duddington A, Collingdon M and Gardner C, 'Dance-Mime: A Contribution to Treatment in Psychiatry'. *Journal of Mental Science*, 99, 308–314, 1953.

Bakali JV, Baldwin SA and Lorentzen S, 'Modelling Group Process Constructs at Three Stages in Group Psychotherapy'. *Psychotherapy Research*, 19 (3), 332–343, 2009.

Bickerdike L, Booth A, Wilson PM, Farley K and Wright K. 'Social Prescribing: Less Rhetoric and More Reality. A Systematic Review of the Evidence'. *British Medical Journal*, 7, e013384, 2017. doi:10.1136/bmjopen-2016-013384

Birdwhistell R, *Kinesics and Context*, Philadelphia, PA: University of Pennsylvania Press, 1970.

Blacking J, *Anthropology of the Body*, London: Academic Press, 1977.

Budman S, Soldz S, Demby A, Feldstein M, Springer T and Davis M, 'Cohesion, Alliance, and Outcome in Group Psychotherapy'. *Psychiatry*, 52, 339–350, 1989.

Burlingame G. M., Fuhriman A., and Johnson J. E., 'Cohesion in Group Psychotherapy'. In J. C. Norcross (Ed.), *Psychotherapy Relationships That Work: Therapist Contributions and Responsiveness to Patients* (pp. 71–87). London: Oxford University Press, 2002.

Burlingame GM, Fuhriman AJ and Johnson J, 'Process and Outcome in Group Counselling and Psychotherapy: A Perspective'. In JL Delucia-Waack, DA Gerrity, CR Kalodner and MT Riva (Eds.), *Handbook of Group Counselling and Psychotherapy* (pp. 49–62), Thousand Oaks, CA: Sage Publications, 2004.

Burlingame GM, McClendon DT and Alonso J, 'Group Cohesion'. In JC Norcross (Ed.), *Psychotherapy Relationships That Work* (2nd Edition), New York: Oxford University Press, 2011.

Buse Z, Sarikaya Z and Colucci E, *The Effectiveness of Dance Movement Therapy (DMT) on Reducing Symptoms of Mental Illnesses: A Systematic Review*. Dissertation submitted in partial fulfillment for MSc, London: Queen Mary University, 2017. doi:10.13140/RG.2.2.16998.52808

Chace M, *Marian Chace, her papers*. Kensington, MD: American Dance Therapy Association, 1975.

Chaiklin H (Ed.), *Marian Chace: Her Papers*, American Dance Therapy Association, 1975.

Chodorow J, *Dance Therapy and Depth Psychology: The Moving Imagination*, London: Routledge, 1991.

Choi JN, Price RH and Vinokur AD, 'Self-Efficacy Changes in Groups: Effects of Diversity, Leadership, and Group Climate'. *Journal of Organizational Behaviour*, 24 (4), 357–372, 2003.

Clift S and Camic PN (Eds.), *Oxford Textbook of Creative Arts Health and Wellbeing: International Perspectives on Practice, Policy, and Research*, Oxford: Open University Press, 2015.

Cohen SJ, *The Modem Dance*, Middletown, CT: Wesleyan University Press, 1966.

Condon W, *Linguistic Kinesic Research and Dance Therapy*, Proceedings, 3rd Annual Conference, ADTA, 1969.

Corey G, *Theory and Practice of Group Counselling*, 8th Edition, Belmont, CA: Thomson/Brooks/Cole Publishing, 2012.

Cozolino L, *The Neuroscience of Human Relationships: Attachment and the Developing Social Brain*. New York: Norton & Co, 2006.

Department of Health and Social Care, www.gov.uk/government/news/social-prescribing-schemes-across-england-to-receive-45-million, 2018.

Dinger U and Schauenburg H, 'Effects of Individual Cohesion and Patient Interpersonal Style on Outcome in Psycho-dynamically Oriented Inpatient Group Psychotherapy'. *Psychotherapy Research*, 20 (1), 22–29, 2010.

Doyne EJ, Ossip-Klein DJ, Bowman ED, Osborn KM, McDougall-Wilson IB and Neimeyer RA, 'Running versus Weight Lifting in the Treatment of Depression'. *Journal of Consulting and Clinical Psychology*, 55, 748–754, 1987.

Espenak L, *Dance Therapy — Theory and Application*, Springfield, IL: Charles Thomas, 1981.

Fancourt D, *Arts in Health: Designing and Researching Interventions*, Oxford: Open University Press, 2017.

Foster J, *The Influences of Rudolf Laban*, London: Lepus Books, 1977.

Gallese V, Keysers C and Rizzolatti G, 'A Unifying View of the Basis of Social Cognition'. *Trends in Cognitive Science*, 8 (9), 396–403, 2004.

Gallese V and Sinigaglia C, 'How the Body in Action Shapes the Self'. *Journal of Consciousness Studies*, 18 (7–8), 117–143, 2011a.

Gallese V and Sinigaglia C, 'What Is so Special about Embodied Simulation?' *Trends in Cognitive Neuroscience*, 15 (11), 512–519, 2011b.

Gendlin E, *Experiencing and the Creation of Meaning*, Glencoe, IL: New York Free Press, 1962.

Gomes N, Menezes MA and Oliveira C, 'Dance Therapy in Patients with Chronic Heart Failure: A Systematic Review and a Meta-Analysis'. *Clinical Rehabilitation*, 28 (12), 1172–9., 2014. doi:10.1177/0269215514534089

Gulbenkian Foundation, *Dance Education and Training in Britain*. (ed. P Brinson), London, 1980.

Hall ET, *The Silent Language*, New York: Doubleday Press, 1973.

Harel Y, Shechtman Z and Cutrona C, 'Individual and Group Process Variables that Affect Social Support in Counselling Groups'. *Group Dynamics: Theory, Research, and Practice*, 15 (4), 297–310, 2011.

Heinicke C and Westheimer I, *Brief Separations*, London: Longman, 1966.

Hendricks G and Wills K, *The Centering Book*, Englewood Cliffs, NJ: Spectrum Books, Prentice-Hall, 1975.

Hornsey MJ, Dwyer L and Oei TPS, 'Beyond Cohesiveness: Reconceptualizing the Link between Group Processes and Outcomes in Group Psychotherapy'. *Small Group Research*, 38 (5), 567–592, 2007.

Horvath AO, 'The Alliance in Context: Accomplishments, Challenges, and Future Directions'. *Psychotherapy: Theory, Research, Practice, Training*, 43 (3), 258–263, 2006.

Hutchinson A, *Labanotation: The System of Analysing and Recording Movement*, Second Edition, London: Oxford University Press, 1970.

Janis I, *Groupthink: Psychological Studies of Policy Decisions and Fiascoes*, Boston, MA: Houghton Muffin, 1982.

Johnson DW and Johnson FP, *Joining Together: Group Theory and Group Skills*, 11th Edition, Harlow, UK: Pearson Education Ltd, 2013.

Johnson JE, Burlingame GM, Olsen JA, Davies DR and Gleave RL, 'Group Climate, Cohesion, Alliance, and Empathy in Group Psychotherapy: Multilevel Structural Equation Models'. *Journal of Counseling Psychology*, 52, 310–321, 2005.

Johnson JE, Pulsipher D, Ferrin SL and Burlingame GM, 'Measuring Group Processes: A Comparison of the GCQ and CCI''. *Group Dynamics: Theory, Research, and Practice*, 10 (2), 136–145, 2006.

Karkou V and Meekums B, 'Dance Movement Therapy for Dementia'. *Cochrane Database of Systematic Reviews*, 3, Art. No.: CD011022, 2014. doi:10.1002/14651858.CD011022

Keleman S, *Your Body Speaks Its Mind*, Berkeley, CA: Center Press, 1981.

Kivlighan DM and Tarrant JM, 'Does Group Climate Mediate the Group Leadership-Group Member Outcome Relationship? A Test of Yalom's Hypotheses about Leadership Priorities'. *Group Dynamics: Theory, Research, and Practice*, 5 (3), 220–234, 2001.

Koch S and Brauninger I, *Advances in Dance/Movement Therapy: Theoretical Perspectives and Empirical Findings*, Berlin: Logos Verlag, 2006.

Koch S, Kuntz T, Lykou S and Cruz R, 'Effects of Dance Movement Therapy and Dance on Health-Related Psychological Outcomes: A Meta-Analysis'. *Arts in Psychotherapy*, 1, 46–64, 2014.

Laban R, *The Mastery of Movement, Revised and Enlarged by Lisa Ullmann*, Third Edition, London: MacDonald and Evans, 1971.

Laban R, *Modern Educational Dance*, revised by Lisa Ullman, third edition, Plymouth: Macdonald & Evans, 1975.

Laban R, 'Some Notes on Movement Therapy'. *Laban Guild Magazine*, 71, 19–20, 1983.

Lamb W and Watson E, *Body Code: The Meaning in Movement*, London: Routledge & Kegan Paul, 1979.

Leste A and Rust J, 'Effects of Dance on Anxiety'. *Journal of Perceptual and Motor Skills*, 58, 767–772, 1984.

Levete G, *No Handicap to Dance*, London: Souvenir Press, 1985.

MacKenzie KR, *Time-Managed Group Psychotherapy: Effective Clinical Applications*, Washington, DC: American Psychiatric Press, 1997.

MacKenzie KR and Livesley WJ, 'A Developmental Model for Brief Group Therapy'. In RR Dies and KR MacKenzie (Eds.), *Advances in Group Psychotherapy: Integrating Research and Practice* (pp. 101–116), New York: International Universities Press, 1983.

Marmarosh CL and Van Horn SM, 'Cohesion in Counselling and Psychotherapy Groups'. In RK Conyne (Ed.), *The Oxford Handbook of Group Counselling* (pp. 137–163), Oxford: Oxford University Press, 2010.

May P, Wexler M, Falkin J and Schoop T, 'Non-verbal Techniques in the Reestablishment of Body Image and Self-id-entity – A Report'. In MN Costonis (Ed.), *Therapy in Motion*. Chicago, IL: University of Illinois Press, 1978.

Meekums B, 'Family Dance Therapy'. *New Dance*, 41, 6–8, 1987.

Meekums B, *Dance Movement Therapy*, London: Sage, 2002.

Meekums B, Karkou V and Nelson EA, 'Dance Movement Therapy for Depression'. *Cochrane Database of Systematic Reviews*, 6, Art. No.: CD009895, 2012. doi:10.1002/14651858.CD009895

Moore CL, *The Harmonic Structure of Movement, Music and Dance according to Rudolf Laban: An Examination of His Unpublished Writings and Drawings*, Lewiston, NY: Edwin Mellen Press Ltd, 2009.

Murcia CQ, Kreutz G, Clift S and Bongard S, 'Shall We Dance? An Exploration of the Perceived Benefits of Dancing on Wellbeing'. *Arts in Health*, 2, 149–163, 2010.

Newlove B, *Laban for Actors and Dancers: Putting Laban's Movement Theory into Practice – A Step-by-Step Guide*, New York: Nick Hern Books. Reprint edition, 1993.

North M, *Personality Assessment Through Movement*, Plymouth: Macdonald & Evans, 1972.

Ogrodniczuk JS and Piper WE, 'The Effect of Group Climate on Outcome in Two Forms of Short-Term Group Therapy'. *Group Dynamics: Theory, Research, and Practice*, 7 (1), 64–76, 2003.

Oliver N, 'Recreation for the Severely Mentally Handicapped', *Proceedings Third Symposium of the Joseph P. Kennedy Jnr. Foundation, Boston, Expanding Concepts in Mental Retardation*, 1968.

Oliver N, 'Physical Activity and the Psychological Development of the Handicapped'. In JE Kane (Ed.), *Psychological Aspects of Physical Education and Sport*, London: Routledge & Kegan Paul, 1975.

Pallaro P (Ed.), *Authentic Movement: Essays by Mary Starks Whitehouse, Janet Adler and Joan Chodorow*, volume one, London: Jessica Kingsley Publishers, 1999.

Pallaro P (Ed.), *Authentic Movement: Moving the Body, Moving the Self, Being Moved. A Collection of Essays*, volume two, London: Jessica Kingsley Publishers, 2007.

Payne H, 'Movement Therapy in a Special Educational Setting', *Cambridge Institute of Education, Conference Proceedings — Current Developments in Special Education*, 1979.

Payne H, 'Movement therapy for the special child'. *British Journal of Dramatherapy*, 4, 3, 1981.

Payne H, 'The Development of the Association for Dance Movement Therapy'. *New Dance*, 27, 17–19, 1983.

Payne H, 'Responding with Dance'. *Maladjustment and Therapeutic Education*, 2 (2), 42–57, 1984.

Payne H, 'Jumping for Joy'. *Changes — Journal for Psychology and Psychotherapy*, 3, 3, 1985.

Payne H, 'The Use of Dance Movement Therapy with Troubled Youth'. In CE Schaefer (Ed.), *Innovative Interventions in Child and Adolescent Therapy*, New York: John Wiley, 1988.

Payne H (Ed.), *Dance Movement Therapy: Theory and Practice*, London: Tavistock/Routledge, 1992.

Payne H (Ed.), *Dance Movement Therapy: Theory, Research and Practice*, London: Routledge, 2006a.

Payne H, 'The Body and Container and Expresser: Authentic Movement Groups in the Development of Wellbeing in Our BodyMindSpirit'. In J Corrigall, H Payne and H Wilkinson (Eds.), *About a Body: Working with the Embodied Mind in Psychotherapy*, London: Routledge, 2006b.

Payne H (Ed.), *Supervision of Dance Movement Psychotherapy: A Practitioner's Handbook*, London/New York: Routledge, 2008.

Payne H, 'The Psycho-neurology of Embodiment with Examples from Authentic Movement and Laban Movement Analysis'. *American Journal of Dance Therapy*, 2017a. doi:10.1007/s10465-017-9256-2

Payne H, 'Introduction: Experiencing Inter-Corporeality and Professional Learning'. In H Payne (Ed.), *Essentials of Dance Movement Psychotherapy: International Perspectives of Theory, Research and Practice*, London/New York: Routledge, 2017b.

Piaget J, *Origins of Intelligence in Childhood*, London: Routledge & Kegan Paul, 1952.

Pirsig RM, *Zen and the Art of Motorcycle Maintenance*, London: Corgi, 1976.

Puretz SL, 'Influence of Modern Dance on Body Image'. In *Essays in Dance Research, Dance Research Annual, IX* (pp. 13–30), New York: CORD, 1978.

Rocha P, Aguiar L, McClelland JA and Morris ME, 'Dance Therapy for Parkinson's Disease: A Randomised Feasibility Study'. *International Journal of Therapy and Rehabilitation*, 25 (2), 2018. doi:10.12968/ijtr.2018.25.2.64

Rogers C, *On Becoming a Person: A Therapist's View of Psychotherapy*. London: Constable, 1967.

Rogers C, *Encounter Groups*, London: Harper Collins, 1970.

Röhricht F and Priebe S, 'Effect of Body-Oriented Psychological Therapy on Negative Symptoms in Schizophrenia: A Randomized Controlled Trial'. *Psychological Medicine*, 36 (5), 669–678, 2006.

Sachs C, *The World History of Dance*, New York: Norton and Co, 1937.

Samaritter R and Payne H, 'Through the Kinaesthetic Lens: Observation of Social Attunement in Autism Spectrum Disorders'. *Behavioural Sciences*, 7, 14, 2017. doi:10.3390/bs7010014

Sandle JN, 'Aesthetics and the Psychology of Qualitative Movement'. In JE Kane (Ed.), *Psychological Aspects of Physical Education and Sport*, London: Routledge & Kegan Paul, 1975.

Schilder P, *The Image and Appearance of the Human Body*, New York: International Universities Press, 1950.

Scholgler B and Trevarthen C, 'To Sing and Dance Together. From Infants to Jazz'. In S Braten (Ed.), *On Being Moved: From Mirror Neurons to Empathy*, Amsterdam: John Bejamins, 2007.

Schoop T, *Won't You Join the Dance?* Palo Alto, CA: Mayfield Publishers, 1973.

Schore A, *The Science of the Art of Psychotherapy*, New York: Norton, 2012.

Shapiro L, *Embodied Cognition*, London: Routledge, 2011.

Sherborne V, 'Building Relationships through Movement with Children with Communication Problems'. *Inscape*, 1, 10, 1974.

Sherborne V, *Developmental Movement for Children*, Second Revised Edition, London: Worth Publishing, 2001.

Siegel DJ, *The Developing Mind: How Human Relationships and the Brain Interact to Shape Who We Are*, Second Edition, New York: Guilford Press, 2012.

Stern D, *The First Relationship — Infant and Mother*, London: Fontana/Open Books, 1979.

Stickley T and Clift S (Eds.), *Arts, Health and Wellbeing: A Theoretical Inquiry for Practice*, Cambridge: Cambridge Scholars Publishing, 2017.

Tarr B, Launay J and Dunbar RIM, 'Silent Disco: Dancing in Synchrony Leads to Elevated Pain Thresholds and Social Closeness'. *Evolutionary Human Behaviour*, 37, 343–349, 2016.

Trevarthen C, 'Neuroscience and Intrinsic Dynamics: Current Knowledge and Potential for Therapy'. In J Corrigall and H Wilkinson (Eds.), *Revolutionary Connections. Psychotherapy and Neuroscience*, London: Routledge, 2003.

Trevarthen C and Delafield-Butt JT, 'Autism as a Developmental Disorder in Intentional Movement and Affective Engagement'. *Frontiers in Integrative Neuroscience*, 7, 49, 2013. doi:10.3389/fnint.2013.00049

Tuckman BW, 'Developmental Sequence in Small Groups'. *Psychological Bulletin*, 63 (6), 384–399, 1965.

Tuckman BW and Jensen MAC, 'Stages of Small-Group Development Revisited'. *Group Facilitation: A Research & Application Journal*, 10 (1), 43–48, 2010.

Wethered A, *Drama and Movement in Therapy*, London: Macdonald & Evans, 1973.

Wethered A and Gardner C, 'Chapter'. In L Burr (Ed.), *Therapy through Movement*, Nottingham: Nottingham Rehabilitation, 1986.

Winnicott DW, *Playing and Reality*, London: Penguin Tavistock Publications, 1971.

Yalom ID and Leszcz M (Collaborator), *The Theory and Practice of Group Psychotherapy* (5th Edition), New York: Basic Books, 2005.